ESSENTIAL IMMUNOLOGY

Essential Immunology

IVAN M. ROITT

MA, DSc(Oxon), FIRCPath

*Professor and Head of Department of Immunology,
Middlesex Hospital Medical School, London W1*

SECOND EDITION

BLACKWELL SCIENTIFIC PUBLICATIONS

OXFORD LONDON EDINBURGH MELBOURNE

© 1971, 1974 by Blackwell Scientific Publications
Osney Mead, Oxford, England
3 Nottingham Street, London W1, England
9 Forrest Road, Edinburgh, Scotland
P.O. Box 9, North Balwyn, Victoria, Australia

ISBN 0 632 00591 2

First published 1971
Reprinted 1972 (twice), 1973 (twice)
Second edition 1974

Spanish edition 1972
Italian edition 1973
German and Portuguese
editions in preparation

Printed and bound in Great Britain by
William Clowes & Sons, Limited, London, Beccles and Colchester

TO MY FAMILY

Contents

viii

9 Autoimmunity   211

Appendix

Acknowledgements

First edition

While not wishing to saddle my colleagues with responsibility for some of the wilder views expressed in this book it would be ungrateful of me not to acknowledge with pleasure the helpful discussions I have had with Jonathan Brostoff, George Dick, Deborah Doniach, Frank Hay, Leslie Hudson, Gerald Jones and John Playfair. I would like to express my appreciation to my secretary, Gladys Stead, who helped to prepare and assemble the manuscript with her usual impeccable expertise and who always encouraged me when my authorship seemed to be faltering. I also wish to acknowledge my debt to Valerie Petts for her excellent help with the photographs. My thanks also to the many people who supplied material for the illustrations; they are acknowledged at the appropriate place in the text. In particular, Bill Weigle kindly let me have unpublished information. Finally let me say that the pain of converting blank paper to written manuscript at home was made bearable by the loving support and understanding of my wife and family.

Second edition

The necessity for a second edition has been dictated by the breakneck increase in immunological knowledge since this book was first written—clearly the subject has too many adherents! My colleagues will know how much I have appreciated their invaluable discussions; particularly I must mention Ita Askonas, Jonathan Brostoff, Deborah Doniach, Arnold Greenberg, Hilliard Festenstein, Frank Hay, Leslie Hudson, D. L. Brown, John Playfair and Mac Turner. Once again I would have been lost without the admirable help of my secretary, Gladys Stead. Even the publishers have been nice!

1 Introduction

Memory, specificity and the recognition of 'non-self'—these lie at the heart of immunology. Our experience of the subsequent protection (*immunity*) afforded by exposure to many infectious illnesses can in fact lead us to this view.

We rarely suffer twice from such diseases as measles, mumps, chicken-pox, whooping cough and so forth. The first contact with an infectious organism clearly imprints some information, imparts some *memory*, so that the body is effectively prepared to repel any later invasion by that organism. This protection is provided by antibodies evoked as a response to the infectious agent behaving as an antigen (figure 1.1). Combination with antibody leads to elimination of the antigen.

By following the production of antibody on the first and second contacts with antigen we can see the basis for the development of immunity. For example, when we inject a bacterial product such as staphylococcal toxoid into a rabbit, several days elapse before antibodies can be detected in the blood; these reach a peak and then fall (figure 1.2). If we now allow the animal to rest and then give a second injection of toxoid, the course of events is dramatically altered. Within two to three days the antibody level in the blood rises steeply to reach much higher values than were observed in the *primary response*. This *secondary response* then is characterized by a more rapid and more abundant production of antibody resulting from the 'tuning up' or priming of the antibody-forming system to provide a population of memory cells after first exposure to antigen.

Vaccination utilizes this principle by employing a relatively harmless form of the antigen (e.g. a killed virus) as the primary stimulus to imprint 'memory'. The body's defences are thereby alerted and any subsequent contact with the virulent form of the organism will lead to a secondary response with an early and explosive production of antibody which will usually prevent the infection from taking hold.

Specificity was mentioned earlier as a fundamental feature of the immunological response. The establishment of memory or

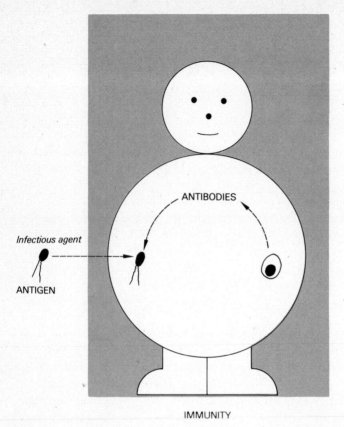

IMMUNITY

FIGURE 1.1. Antibodies (*anti*-foreign *bodies*) are produced by host white cells on contact with the invading micro-organism which is acting as an antigen (i.e. *gen*erates *anti*bodies). The individual may then be immune to further attacks.

immunity by one organism does not confer protection against another unrelated organism. After an attack of measles we are immune to further infection but are susceptible to other agents such as the polio or mumps viruses. The body can, in fact, differentiate specifically between the two organisms.

This ability to recognize one antigen and distinguish it from another goes even further. The individual must also recognize what is foreign, i.e. what is '*non-self*'. The failure to discriminate between 'self' and 'non-self' could lead to the synthesis of antibodies directed against components of the subject's own body (*autoantibodies*) which in principle could prove to be highly embarrassing. On purely theoretical grounds it seemed to Burnet and Fenner that the body must develop some mechanism whereby 'self' and 'non-self' could be distin-

2

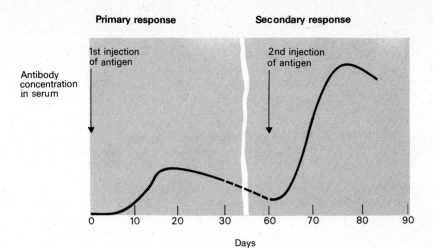

FIGURE 1.2. *Primary and secondary response*. A rabbit is injected on two separate occasions with staphylococcal toxoid. The antibody response on the second contact with antigen is more rapid and more intense.

guished, and they postulated that those circulating body components which were able to reach the developing lymphoid system in the perinatal period could in some way be 'learnt' as 'self'. A permanent unresponsiveness or tolerance would then be created so that as immunological maturity were reached there would be an inability to respond to 'self' components. As we shall see later, these predictions have been amply verified.

It is worth emphasizing that the lower animal forms possess so-called 'non-specific immunity' mechanisms such as phago-cytosis of bacteria by specialized cells, which afford them pro-tection from infecting organisms. The *adaptive* immune response in higher animals which we have been discussing, has evolved to provide more effective defence in that appropriate immunological cells concentrate their energies on the particular agents infecting the body at any one time and the specific anti-bodies which they synthesize greatly speed up the disposal of these organisms by facilitating their adherence to phagocytic cells (see chapter 7). In other words the specific adaptive immune response operates to a considerable extent by increasing the efficiency of the non-specific immunity systems.

Some historical perspectives

Space does not allow more than a cursory survey of some of the outstanding contributions to the development of immunology.
India and China (ancient times)—Practice of 'variolation' in

3

which protection against smallpox was obtained by inoculating live organisms from disease pustules (dangerous!).

Jenner (1798)—Protective effect of vaccination with non-virulent cowpox against smallpox infection (noting the pretty pox-free skin of the milkmaids).

Pasteur (1881)—Vaccine for anthrax using attenuated organisms.

Metchnikoff (1883)—Role of phagocytes in immunity.

Von Behring (1890)—Recognized antibodies in serum to diphtheria toxin.

Denys & Leclef (1895)—Phagocytosis greatly enhanced by immunization.

Bordet (1899)—Lysis of cells by antibody requires co-operation of serum factors now collectively termed complement.

Landsteiner (1900)—Human ABO groups and natural isohaemagglutinins.

Richet & Portier (1902)—Anaphylaxis (opposite of prophylaxis).

Wright (1903)—Relation of opsonic activity to phagocytosis.

Zinsser (1925)—Contrast between immediate and delayed-type hypersensitivity.

Heidelberger & Kendall (1930–35)—Quantitative precipitin studies on antigen–antibody interactions.

Later work is referred to in subsequent chapters but note in particular the finding that immunization leads to more effective phagocytosis. At this stage we can examine the work of Heidelberger and Kendall and its implications in more detail and with some benefit.

The classical precipitin reaction

When an antigen solution is mixed in correct proportions with a potent antiserum, a precipitate is formed. Quantitative analysis of this interaction by the method shown in figure 1.3 gives both the antibody content of the immune serum and also an indication of the valency of the antigen. This can vary enormously depending on the antigen, its size, and the species making the antibody. With rabbit antisera, ovalbumin may have a valency of 10 and human thyroglobulin as many as 40 combining sites on its surface. By splitting antigens into large fragments with proteolytic enzymes it has become clear that the separate combining areas on the surface of a given protein (called anti-genic *determinants* or *epitopes*) are by no means identical.

It will be noted from the precipitin curve in figure 1.3 that as

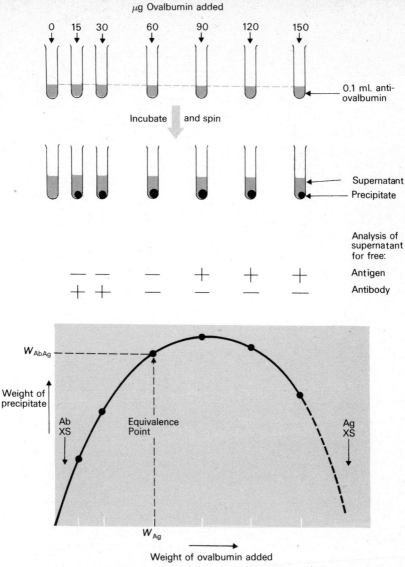

FIGURE 1.3. Quantitative precipitin reaction between rabbit anti-ovalbumin and ovalbumin (after Heidelberger & Kendall). Increasing amounts of ovalbumin are added to a constant volume of the antiserum placed in a number of tubes. After incubation the precipitates formed are spun down and weighed. Each supernatant is split into two halves: by adding antigen to one and antibody to the other, the presence of reactive antibody or antigen respectively can be demonstrated. The antibody content of the serum can be calculated from the equivalence point where no antigen or antibody is present in the supernatant. All the antigen added is therefore complexed in the precipitate with all the antibody available and the antibody content in 0·1 ml of serum would therefore be given by (W_{AgAb}–W_{Ag}). Analysis of the precipitate formed in antibody excess (AbXS), where the antigen-combining sites are largely saturated, gives a measure of the molar ratio of antibody to antigen in the complex and hence an estimate of the antigen valency.

5

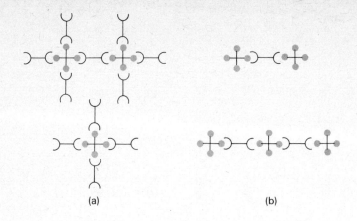

FIGURE 1.4. Diagrammatic representation of complexes formed between a hypothetical tetravalent antigen ($\bullet\mkern-2mu\vert\mkern-2mu\bullet$) and bivalent antibody (>−<)

mixed in different proportions. In practice, the antigen valencies are unlikely to lie in the same plane or to be formed by identical determinants as suggested in the figure.

(a) Complexes in extreme antibody excess. Antigen valencies saturated and molar ratio Ab:Ag approximates to the valency of the antigen.

(b) Complexes in antigen excess. In extreme excess where the two valencies of each antibody molecule become rapidly saturated, the complex Ag_2Ab tends to predominate.

(c) Large three-dimensional lattice obtained in typical immune precipitate.

(d) Monovalent antigen binds but is unable to cross-link antibody molecules.

more and more antigen is added, an optimum is reached after which consistently less precipitate is formed. At this stage the supernatant can be shown to contain soluble complexes of antigen (Ag) and antibody (Ab), many of composition Ag_4Ab_3, Ag_3Ab_2 and Ag_2Ab. In extreme antigen excess (AgXS, figure 1.3) ultracentrifugal analysis reveals the complexes to be mainly of the form Ag_2Ab, suggesting that the rabbit antibodies studied are bivalent (figure 1.4; see also figures 2.6 and 2.7). Between these extremes the crosslinking of antigen and antibody will generally give rise to three-dimensional lattice structures, as suggested by Marrack, which coalesce to form large precipitating aggregates.

The basis of specificity

Much of our understanding of the factors governing antigen specificity has come from the studies of Landsteiner and of Pauling and their colleagues on the interaction of antibody with small chemically defined groupings termed *haptens*, a typical example being *m*-aminobenzene sulphonate (figure 1.5). Whereas an antigen will both evoke antibody formation and combine with the resulting antibody, *a hapten is defined as a small molecule which by itself cannot stimulate antibody synthesis but will combine with antibody once formed.*

   The problem of how to produce these antibodies was solved by coupling the haptens to proteins which acted as 'carriers'. It then became possible to relate variations in the chemical structure of a hapten to its ability to bind to a given antibody. In one experiment, antibodies raised to *m*-aminobenzene sulphonate were tested for their ability to combine with *ortho, meta* and *para* isomers of the hapten and related molecules in which the sulphonate group was substituted by arsonate or carboxylate (figure 1.6). The results are summarized in table 1.1. The hapten with the sulphonate group in the *ortho* position combines somewhat less well with the antibody than the original *meta* isomer, but the *para*-substituted compound (chemically similar to the *ortho*) shows very poor reactivity. The substitution of arsonate for sulphonate leads to weaker combination with the antibody; both groups are negatively charged and have

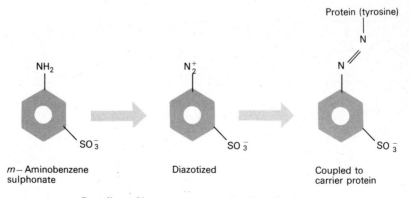

m – Aminobenzene sulphonate

Diazotized

Coupled to carrier protein

FIGURE 1.5. Coupling of hapten to protein by diazotization.

7

TABLE 1.1. Effect of variations in hapten structure on strength of binding to *m*-aminobenzene sulphonate antibodies

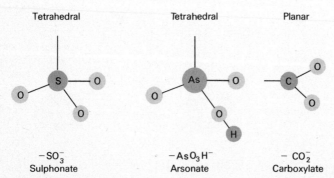

	ortho	*meta*	*para* isomers
R = sulphonate	+ +	+ + +	±
R = arsonate	−	+	−
R = carboxylate	−	±	−

Strength of binding is directly graded from negative (−) to very strong (+ + +). Since free haptens can only combine with one antibody-combining site and cannot therefore cross-link, they form only soluble complexes; their binding strength was assessed through their ability to inhibit precipitation by antibody of a new carrier protein substituted with several of the original hapten (*m*-aminobenzene sulphonate) groups per molecule (from Landsteiner K. & van der Scheer J. *J.exp.Med.* 1936, **63**, 325)

a tetrahedral structure but the arsonate group is larger in size and has an extra H atom (figure 1.6). The aminobenzoates in which the sulphonate is substituted by the negatively charged but planar carboxylate group show even less affinity for the antibody. It would appear that the overall *configuration* of the hapten is even more important than its *chemical* nature, i.e. the hapten is recognized by the overall three-dimensional shape of its outer electron cloud as distinct from its chemical reactivity. The production of antibodies against such strange moieties as benzene sulphonate and arsonate becomes more comprehensible if they are thought to be directed against a particular electron-cloud shape rather than a specific chemical structure. This view is consistent with the nature of antigen–antibody binding which is known not to involve covalent linkages.

FIGURE 1.6. Configurations of the sulphonate, arsonate and carboxylate groups.

It should be stressed immediately that the forces which hold antigen and antibody together are in essence no different from the so-called 'non-specific' protein–protein interactions which occur between any two unrelated proteins (or other macromolecules) as, for example, human serum albumin and human transferrin. These intermolecular forces may be classified under four headings:

(a) *Coulombic*

These are due to the attraction between oppositely charged ionic groups on the two protein side chains as, for example, an ionized amino group (NH_3^+) on a lysine of one protein and an ionized carboxyl group ($-COO^-$) of, say, aspartate on the other (figure 1.7a). The force of attraction (F) is inversely proportional to the square of the distance (d) between the charges, i.e.

$$F \propto 1/d^2$$

Thus as the charges come closer together, the attractive force increases considerably: if we halve the distance apart, we quadruple the attraction. Dipoles on antigen and antibody can also attract each other. In addition, electrostatic forces may be generated by charge transfer reactions between antibody and antigen; for example an electron-donating protein residue such as tryptophan could part with an electron to a group such as dinitrophenyl which is electron-accepting thereby creating an effective $+1$ charge on the antibody and -1 on the antigen.

(b) *Hydrogen bonding*

The formation of the relatively weak and reversible hydrogen bridges between hydrophilic groups such as .OH, .NH_2 and .COOH depends very much upon the close approach of the two molecules carrying these groups (figure 1.7b).

(c) *Hydrophobic*

The side chains of amino acids such as valine, leucine and phenylalanine are hydrophobic ('water-hating') and in aqueous solution, the water molecules with which they come into contact are not H-bonded and are therefore in a higher energy

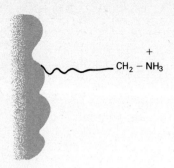
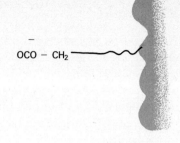

Lysine
side – chain

Aspartate
side – chain

(a)

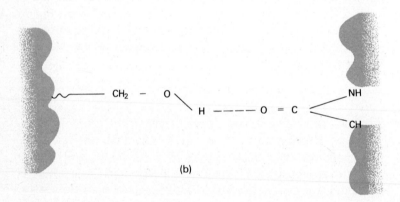

(b)

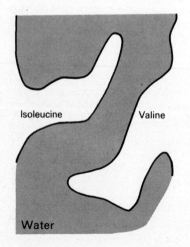
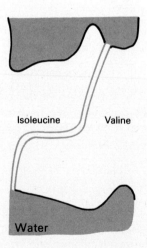

Isoleucine   Valine

Isoleucine   Valine

Water

Water

(c)

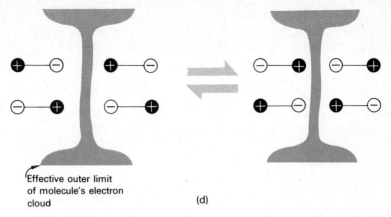

Effective outer limit
of molecule's electron
cloud

(d)

FIGURE 1.7. Protein–protein interactions.

(a) Coulombic attraction between oppositely charged ionic groupings.

(b) Hydrogen bonding between two proteins: the examples shows a H-bond between a serine or threonine side chain on one protein and a peptide carbonyl group on the other.

(c) Hydrophobic bonding: the region in which the water molecules are not hydrogen bonded because of contact with the hydrophobic groups (indicated by the thickened line) is considerably reduced when the hydrophobic groups on two proteins are in contact with each other. More water molecules are now in the H-bonded state and the lower free-energy of this system makes this a more probable state than separation of the hydrophobic groups.

(d) Van der Waals forces: the interaction between the electrons in the external orbitals of two different macromolecules may be envisaged (for simplicity!) as the attraction between induced oscillating dipoles in the two electron clouds.

state than they would be if free to form more hydrogen bonds with themselves or some hydrophilic molecule. If hydrophobic groups on the surfaces of two proteins come into close contact so as to exclude water molecules between them, the net surface in contact with water is reduced (figure 1.7c). Thus more water molecules are in the H-bonded state than when the two proteins are apart: this means that the proteins take up a lower energy state and hence a preferred configuration when they are combined rather than separated (in other words, there is a force of attraction between them). It has been estimated that hydrophobic forces may contribute up to 50% of the total strength of the antigen-antibody bond.

(d) *Van der Waals*

These are the forces between molecules which depend upon interaction between the external 'electron clouds'. The deviation of gaseous molecules of say nitrogen or hydrogen from 'ideal' behaviour according to the kinetic theory is attributable to the Van der Waals attractions between them. The nature of this interaction is difficult to describe in non-mathematical terms but it has been likened to a temporary perturbation of electrons in one molecule effectively forming a dipole which induces a dipolar perturbation in the other molecule, the two dipoles then having a force of attraction between them; as the displaced electrons swing back through the equilibrium position and beyond, the dipoles oscillate (figure 1.7d). The force of attraction is inversely proportional to the seventh power of the distance, i.e.

$$F \propto 1/d^7$$

and as a result this rises very rapidly as the interacting molecules come closer together.

This last point underlines one essential feature common to all four types of force—they depend upon the close approach of both molecules before the forces become of significant magnitude. And this is at the heart of the combination of antigen and antibody. By having *complementary* electron-cloud shapes on the combining site of the antibody and the surface determinant of the antigen, the two molecules can fit snugly together like a lock and key (figure 1.9a). The intermolecular distance becomes very small and the 'non-specific protein interaction forces' are considerably increased; the greater the areas of antigen and antibody which fit together, the greater the force of attraction, particularly if there is apposition of opposite charges and hydrophobic groupings.

ANTIBODY AFFINITY

The combination of antibody with the surface determinant of an antigen or a monovalent hapten molecule (cf. figure 1.4d) is reversible and the complex may readily dissociate, depending upon the strength of binding. This can be defined through the equilibrium constant (K) of the reaction:

$$Ab + Hp \rightleftharpoons AbHp$$

$$(\supset\!\!\!-\!\!\!\subset) \quad (\,\bullet\,) \quad (\supset\!\!\!-\!\!\!-\!\!\!(\bullet))$$

given by the mass action equation,

$$K = \frac{[AbHp]}{[Ab][Hp]}$$

where [Ab] is the concentration of antibody combining sites and [Hp] the concentration of hapten. If the antibody and

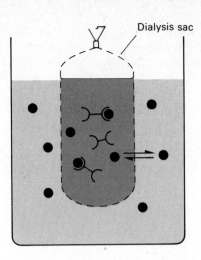

Dialysis sac

FIGURE 1.8. Antibody affinity determined by studying the equilibrium between antibody (⊃⊂) and hapten (●). Within the dialysis sac the hapten is partly in the free form and partly bound to antibody according to the affinity of the antibody. Only hapten can diffuse through the dialysis membrane and the external concentration then will equal the concentration of unbound hapten within the sac. Measurement of total hapten in the dialysis sac then enables the amount bound to antibody to be calculated. By repeating this at different concentrations of hapten, one can calculate the average affinity constant (K) as described in the text. Constant renewal of the external buffer will lead to total dissociation and loss of hapten from inside the dialysis sac showing the reversible nature of the antigen–antibody bond.

hapten fit together very closely, the equilibrium will lie well over to the right; we refer to such antibodies which bind strongly to the hapten as *high affinity antibodies*. At a certain *free* hapten concentration $[Hp_c]$ where half of the antibody sites are bound, $[AbHp] = [Ab]$ and $K = 1/[Hp_c]$, i.e. K is equal to the reciprocal of the concentration of free hapten at the equilibrium point where half the antibody sites are in the bound form. In other words, when an antibody has a high affinity constant and binds hapten strongly, it only needs a low hapten concentration to half-saturate the antibody. Affinity constants, which can be determined by methods such as that shown in figure 1.8, may reach values as high as 10^{10} litres/mole.

Analysis of the binding at different hapten concentrations generally shows a heterogeneity which indicates that most antisera, even those raised against antigens with a simple structure, contain a variety of different antibodies with a range of binding affinities which depend upon the area of contact between the antibody and the antigenic determinant, the closeness of fit (figure 1.9) and the distribution of charged and

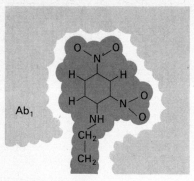

(a) High affinity

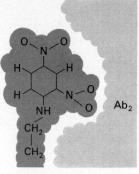

(b) Moderate affinity

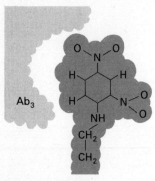

(c) Low affinity

FIGURE 1.9. Binding of antibodies present in the same antiserum with different affinities to the same hapten (dinitrobenzene linked to the amino group of lysine).

(a) Antibody$_1$ fits with nearly the whole of the hapten and is thus of high affinity.

(b) Antibody$_2$ fits with less of the molecule and not so closely, and has a moderate binding affinity while (c) the low affinity antibody$_3$ is complementary in shape to so little of the hapten surface that its binding energy is very little above that occurring between completely unrelated proteins. Only a portion of the antibody combining site is shown.

hydrophobic groups. If we bear in mind that antigen determinants are not two-dimensional as represented in the figures, but have a three-dimensional electron-cloud shape, one can realize that antibodies are confronted with very many different configurations even in a single determinant, depending upon the direction from which the antibody molecule approaches. Another factor should be considered; antibody molecules may be able to adapt themselves to the shape of the antigen determinant to some extent and Kabat has drawn attention to the exceptional number of glycines near to the combining region which could impart a high degree of flexibility to the structure.

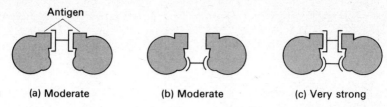

Antigen

(a) Moderate   (b) Moderate   (c) Very strong

FIGURE 1.10. The 'bonus' effect of multivalent attachment on binding strength. The force binding the two antigen molecules in (c) with two antibody bridges is often at least 10 times greater than (a+b) where only single antibody molecules provide the link. The effect varies with K values; the weaker the affinity the more the bonus.

AVIDITY AND THE BONUS EFFECT OF
MULTIVALENT BINDING

The strength of the interaction of antibody with a monovalent hapten or a single antigen determinant we have labelled antibody affinity. In most practical situations we are concerned with the interaction of an antiserum with a full antigen molecule and the term employed to express this binding,

$$n\text{Ab} + m\text{Ag} \rightleftharpoons \text{Ab}_n\text{Ag}_m$$

is *avidity*. The factors which contribute to avidity are complicated. Not only must we contend with the heterogeneity of antibodies in a given serum which are directed against a single determinant on the antigen, but we must also recognize that the differing amino acid sequences on different parts of a protein surface, for example, lead to the formation of a number of antigenic patches or determinants on a single molecule, each with its distinct shape and specificity.

The multivalence of most antigens leads to an interesting 'bonus' effect in which the binding of two antigen molecules by antibody is always greater than the arithmetic sum of the individual antibody links. This is illustrated in figure 1.10. The mechanism of this effect may be interpreted by considering an analogy. Let us fabricate an unheard of disease in which we cannot stop our hands opening and closing continuously. If we now try to hold an object in *one* hand it will fall the moment we open that hand. However, if we use *both* hands to hold the object, provided we open and close our hands at different times, there is much less chance of the object falling. The reversible combination of antigen and antibody is like the opening and closing of the hand; the more valencies holding the antigen the less likely it is to be lost when the complex dissociates at any one binding site (figure 1.11).

15

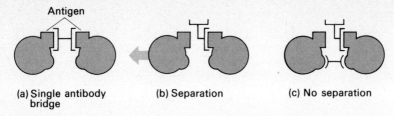

(a) Single antibody   (b) Separation   (c) No separation
bridge

FIGURE I.II. The mechanism of the bonus effect. Each antigen–antibody
bond is reversible and with a single antibody bridge between two antigen
molecules (a), dissociation of either bond could enable an antigen molecule
to 'escape' as in (b). If there are two antibody bridges, even when one
dissociates the other prevents the antigen molecule from escaping and holds
it in position ready to reform the broken bond.

SPECIFICITY AND CROSS-REACTIONS

An antiserum raised against a given antigen can cross-react with
a partially related antigen which bears one or more identical or
similar determinants. In figure 1.12 it can be seen that an antiserum to antigen$_1$ will react less strongly with antigen$_2$ which
bears just one identical determinant because only certain of the
antibodies in the serum can bind. Antigen$_3$ which possesses a
similar but not identical determinant will not fit as well with the
antibody and the binding is even weaker. Antigen$_4$ which has
no structural similarity at all will not react significantly with
the antibody.* Thus, based upon stereochemical considerations,
we can see why the avidity of the antiserum for antigens$_{2+3}$ is
less than for the homologous antigen, while for the unrelated
antigen$_4$ it is negligible. It is in this way that the *specificity* of an
antiserum is expressed.

* If the antigenic determinant is appreciably smaller than the antibody site,
there could be a cross-reaction with an unrelated antigen which bound
fortuitously to the remainder of the site.

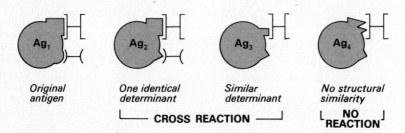

Original   One identical   Similar   No structural
antigen   determinant   determinant   similarity

└─── CROSS REACTION ───┘   └─ NO REACTION ─┘

FIGURE I.12. Specificity and cross-reaction. The avidity of the serum
(antibodies ⊢ , ⊣⊂) for $Ag_1 > Ag_2 > Ag_3 \gg Ag_4$ so that the serum
shows specificity.

The forces which bind antigen to antibody are largely similar to those binding enzyme to substrate. The elucidation of the three-dimensional structures of certain enzymes such as lysozyme by X-ray crystallography has shown that the substrate lies within a long cleft in the surface of the molecule. Similar studies on homogeneous antibody preparations indicate that the combining site is probably a relatively flat area, about 25×20 A, which includes a shallow groove 15×6 with a depth of 6 A, and has a number of protruding side chains (Poljak and colleagues).

These dimensions are consistent with studies using linear haptens formed from repeating units of sugar molecules (Kabat) or amino acids (Sela) which have indicated that the site probably accommodates roughly six such units. Of these units, the terminal one usually shows the highest binding energy to the antibody and may be termed the 'immunodominant' group; successive units contribute progressively less to the overall binding. Recent investigations by Benjamini into tobacco mosaic virus (TMV) protein and its antibodies have shown firstly that the C-terminal decapeptide has strong antibody-binding activity (figure 1.13a) and surprisingly, the antibody has a comparable affinity for the C-terminal tripeptide coupled with an octanoyl (hydrophobic) group at the N-terminal end (figure 1.13b). It would appear that the major contribution to specificity is made by the configuration of the three terminal amino acid residues, and that a further significant factor in the binding energy is derived from non-specific interaction with hydrophobic groupings further back in the antibody site. It will be of importance to know whether these results hold true for other antigens.

So far we have discussed the interaction of linear antigens with the antibody combining site. A different situation arises with globular proteins and as might be expected the main antigenic determinants are located on those portions of the polypeptide chain which protrude as angular bends capable of

(a) H_2N—Thr.Thr.Ala.Glu.Thr.Leu.Asp.Ala.Arg.COOH

(b) $CH_3(CH_2)_6CO$—Asp.Ala.Arg.COOH

FIGURE 1.13. The C-terminal decapeptide of TMV protein (a) and the octanoyl derivative of the C-terminal tripeptide (b) which have comparable antibody-binding activities.

lying within an antibody cleft as was established with myoglobin for example. The linear *sequence* of amino acids in the peptide chain is clearly important for specificity but the overall *conformation* of the peptide makes a very significant contribution to the energy of binding with antibody. Lysozyme provides a case in point: this protein has an intrachain-disulphide bond which forms a loop in the peptide chain. As Arnon has shown, certain antibodies reacting with lysozyme can be inhibited by prior addition of the isolated loop peptide. However, reduction of the disulphide bond destroys this inhibitory activity even though the linear chain so formed has an unchanged primary amino acid sequence.

It is worth emphasizing that our analysis has been concerned with the interaction of an antigenic determinant or a hapten with antibody but several further factors govern the ability of a given substance to act as an *antigen*, i.e. to stimulate the antigen-reactive cells in the host animal to produce antibody (cf chapter 3).

Further reading

Davis B.D., Dulbecco R., Eisen H.N., Ginsberg H.S. & Wood W.B. (1968) *Principles of Microbiology and Immunology*. Harper International Edition.
Kabat E.A. (1968) *Structural Concepts in Immunology and Immunochemistry*. Holt, Rinehart & Winston Inc, New York.
Good R.A. & Fisher D.W. (eds.) (1972) *Immunobiology*. Sinauer Associates Ltd, Stamford, Conn.
Bellanti J.A. (1971) *Immunology*. W.B. Saunders, Philadelphia.
Day E.D. (1972) *Advanced Immunochemistry*. Williams & Wilkins, Baltimore.
Brent L. & Holborow E. J. (eds) (1974) *Progress in Immunology*. North Holland, Amsterdam. (Papers from the 2nd Int. Congress of Immunology).
Rose N.R., Milgrom F. & van Oss C.J. (eds) (1973) *Principles of Immunology*. Macmillan, New York.

Historical

Parish H.J. (1968) *Victory with Vaccines*. Livingstone, Edinburgh.
Landsteiner K. (1946) *The Specificity of Serological Reactions*. Harvard University Press (reprinted 1962 by Dover Publications, New York).

Series for the advanced student

Advances in Immunology (Annual). Academic Press, London.
Perspectives in Immunology (Brook Lodge Symposia). Academic Press, London.
Progress in Allergy. S. Karger, Basle.
Modern Trends in Immunology. Butterworths, London.
Transplantation Reviews (ed. G. Moller). Munksgaard, Copenhagen.
Essays in Fundamental Immunology. Blackwell Scientific Publications, Oxford.

Contemporary Topics in Molecular Immunology. Plenum Press, N.Y.
Contemporary Topics in Immunobiology. Plenum Press, N.Y.
Protides of the Biological Fluids. Pergamon Press, Oxford.

Current information

Current Titles in Immunology, Transplantation & *Allergy*. Sciences, Engineering Medical & Business Data Ltd, Oxford.

Major journals

Nature, Lancet, Science, J.exp.Med., Immunology, J.Immunology, Clin.exp. Immunology, Immunochemistry. Int.Arch.Allergy, Cell.Immunology, European J.Immunology, Scand.J.Immunol., Clin.Immunol & Immunopath., J.Immunogenetics, J.Immunol.Methods. J.Reticuloendoth.Soc., Tissue Antigens.

Special articles

Richards F.F. & Konigsberg W.M. (1973) How specific are antibodies? *Immunochemistry*, **10**, 545.
Sela M. (1969) Antigenicity: some molecular aspects. *Science*, **166**, 1365.

2 The immunoglobulins

The association of antibody activity with the classical γ-globulin fraction of serum was shown many years ago by Tiselius and Kabat. They hyperimmunized rabbits with pneumococcal polysaccharide to produce a high concentration of circulating antibody and then examined the effect of absorbing the serum with antigen on the electrophoretic profile. Only the γ-globulin fraction was significantly reduced after removal of antibody (figure 2.1). With the recognition of heterogeneity in the types of molecules which can function as antibodies, it has now become customary to use the general term 'immunoglobulin'. In each species, the immunoglobulin molecules can be subdivided into different classes on the basis of the structure of their 'backbone' (rather than on their specificity for given antigens). Thus, in the human for example, five major structural types or classes can be distinguished: immunoglobulin G (abbreviated to IgG), IgM, IgA, IgD and IgE.

The basic structure of the immunoglobulins

The antibody fraction of serum consists predominantly of one group of proteins with molecular weight around 150,000 (sedimentation coefficient 7S) of which the major component is IgG, and another of molecular weight 900,000 (19S IgM). The IgG antibodies can be split by papain into three fragments (R.R. Porter). Two of these are identical and are able to combine with

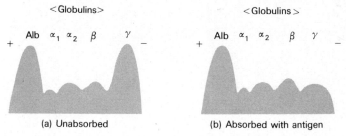

(a) Unabsorbed   (b) Absorbed with antigen

FIGURE 2.1. Association of antibody activity with γ-globulin serum fraction. Hyperimmune serum is separated into major fractions by electrophoresis before (a) and after (b) absorption with antigen. Only the γ-globulin fraction is reduced.

antigen to form a soluble complex which will not precipitate; these are therefore univalent antibody fragments and are given the nomenclature Fab ('fragment antigen binding'). The third fragment has no power to combine with antigen and is termed Fc ('fragment crystallizable' obtainable in crystalline form). Another proteolytic enzyme, pepsin, cleaves the Fc part from the remainder of the antibody molecule, leaving a large fragment ($5S$) which can still precipitate with antigen and is formulated as $F(ab')_2$ since it is clearly still divalent.

Antibodies can also be broken down into their constituent peptide chains. First the disulphide bonds linking different chains must be broken by reduction with *excess* of a sulphydryl reagent (e.g. 2-mercaptoethanol: $HO-CH_2-CH_2-SH$) which drives the following reaction from left to right:

$$
\begin{array}{c}
\overline{} \\
S \\
| \\
S \\
\underline{}
\end{array}
\quad + \quad RSH \quad \rightleftharpoons \quad
\begin{array}{c}
\overline{} \\
SH \\
\\
SH \\
\underline{}
\end{array}
\quad + \quad RS-SR
$$

Cross-linked peptide chains	Excess sulphydryl reagent	Unlinked peptide chains	

The reduced molecule still has a sedimentation coefficient of $7S$ because the chains are held together by non-covalent forces but they can be separated by lowering the pH with acid (G. Edel-

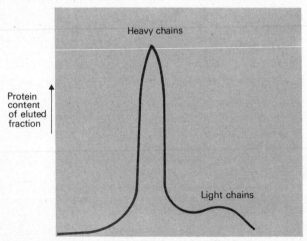

Eluted fractions coming off column.

FIGURE 2.2. Gel filtration of reduced and acidified $7S$ γ-globulin (IgG fraction) on Sephadex G75. The cross-linked dextran Sephadex gel has pores with a variety of sizes. The smaller chains can penetrate more deeply into the gel via the smaller pores than the larger chains which are therefore less retarded on the column and appear first in the effluent (from Fleischman J., Pain R.H. & Porter R.R. *Arch.Bioch.Biophys.* 1962, Suppl. 1, 174).

N-terminal   C-terminal

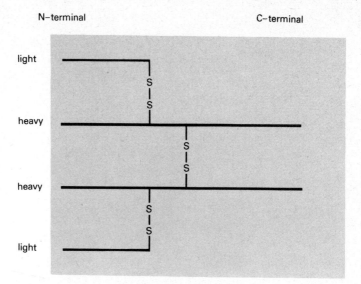

FIGURE 2.3. Antibody model proposed by R.R.Porter with two heavy and two light polypeptide chains held by interchain disulphide bonds. In the diagram the amino-terminal residue is on the left for each chain.

man). Fractionation using gel filtration reveals two sizes of peptide chain termed *light* and *heavy chains* (figure 2.2).

On the basis of these findings Porter put forward a symmetrical four-peptide model for antibody consisting of two heavy and two light chains linked together by interchain disulphide bonds (figure 2.3). The formation of the various fragments by proteolysis and reduction is represented in figure 2.4.

Purified IgG antibodies when visualized in the electron microscope by negative staining can be seen to be Y-shaped molecules whose arms can swing out to an angle of 180° through the papain and pepsin sensitive region acting as a hinge (figure 2.5). Amino acid analysis of the hinge region has revealed an unusual feature—a large number of proline residues; because of its structure, proline prevents the peptide chain assuming α-helix conformation. This stretch of the chain (present in rabbit F(ab′)$_2$ but absent from Fab) of sequence:

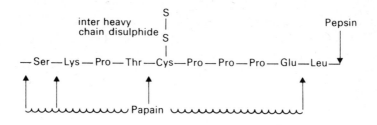

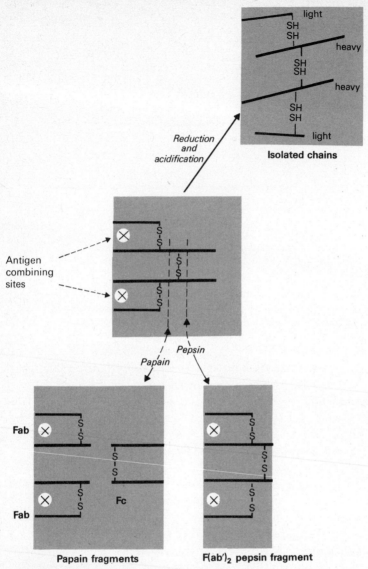

FIGURE 2.4. Degradation of immunoglobulin to constituent peptide chains and to proteolytic fragments showing divalence of pepsin $F(ab')_2$ and univalence of the papain Fab. After pepsin digestion the pFc′ fragment representing the C-terminal half of the Fc region is formed. The portion of the heavy chain in the Fab fragment is given the symbol Fd.

is therefore extended and the peptide links are accessible to the proteolytic enzymes which act at the bonds shown.

Elegant confirmation of the correctness of these general views on the structure of the antibody molecule has come from studies using a divalent hapten, bis-N-dinitrophenyl (DNP)-octamethylene-diamine:

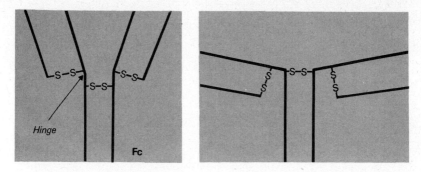

FIGURE 2.5. Illustrating the flexibility of the immunoglobulin molecule at the hinge region. Compare with conformation of immunoglobulin molecules in figure 2.6.

$$NO_2-\bigcirc-NH-CH_2CH_2CH_2CH_2CH_2CH_2CH_2CH_2-NH-\bigcirc-NO_2$$

where the two haptenic DNP groups are far enough apart not to interfere with each other's combination with antibody. When mixed with purified IgG antibody to DNP, the divalent hapten brings the antigen-combining sites on two different antibodies together end to end; when viewed by negative staining in the electron microscope a series of geometric forms are observed which represent the different structures to be expected if a Y-shaped hinged molecule with a combining site at the end of each of the two arms of the Y were to complex with this divalent hapten. Triangular trimers, square tetramers and pentagonal pentamers may be readily discerned (figure 2.6). The way in which these polymeric forms arise is indicated in figure 2.7. The position of the Fc fragment and its lack of involvement in the combination with antigen are apparent from the shape of the polymers formed using the pepsin F(ab')$_2$ fragment (figure 2.6e).

Variations in structure of the immunoglobulins

Any attempt to analyse the amino acid structure of the immunoglobulins in normal serum is bedevilled by the incredible number of different molecules present. This heterogeneity may be inferred from analysis by immunoelectrophoresis, the principle of which is explained in figure 2.8. It is evident that the immunoglobulins occur in different classes of

25

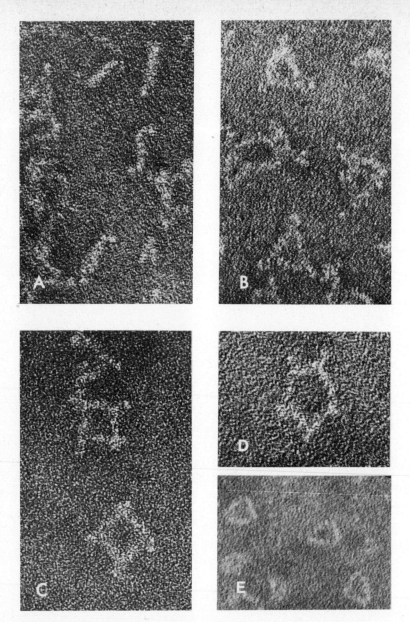

FIGURE 2.6. (a)–(d) Electron micrograph (× 1,000,000) of complexes formed on mixing the divalent DNP hapten with rabbit anti-DNP antibodies. The 'negative stain' phosphotungstic acid is an electron-dense solution which penetrates in the spaces between the protein molecules. Thus the protein stands out as a 'light' structure in the electron beam. The hapten links together the Y-shaped antibody molecules to form (a) dimers, (b) trimers, (c) tetramers and (d) pentamers.

(e) As in (b); trimers formed using the F(ab′)$_2$ antibody fragment from which the Fc structures have been digested by pepsin (× 500,000). The trimers can be seen to lack the Fc projections at each corner evident in (b). (After Valentine R.C. & Green N.M., *J.mol.Biol.* 1967, **27**, 615; courtesy of Dr. Green and with the permission of Acad. Press, N.Y.)

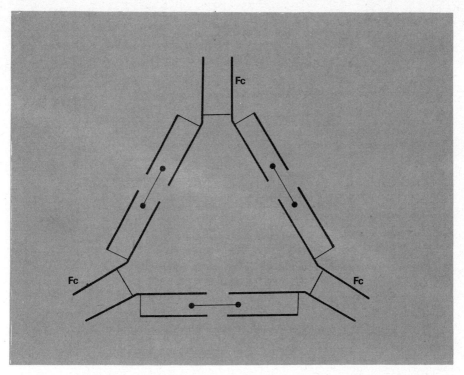

FIGURE 2.7. Three DNP antibody molecules held together as a trimer by the divalent hapten (●————●). Compare figure 2.6b. When the Fc fragments are first removed by pepsin, the corner pieces are no longer visible (figure 2.6e).

molecules and also that they have a very wide range of electrophoretic mobilities within each class, ranging in the case of IgG, from slow γ- to α_2-globulin (figure 2.9). This range of mobilities is due to different net charges on the different immunoglobulin molecules and is indicative of variations in amino acid structure (e.g. replacement of a neutral residue such as valine with a basic amino acid like lysine will tend to increase the net charge by $+1$). Even 'purified' antibodies directed against a simple hapten may show a wide spectrum of electrophoretic mobilities since, as mentioned in the previous chapter, they represent a variety of antibodies of varying degrees of fit for various shapes on the hapten surface.

The answer to this seemingly insoluble problem of analysing amino acid structure has come from study of the *myeloma proteins*. In the human disease known as multiple myeloma, one cell making one particular individual immunoglobulin divides over and over again in the uncontrolled way a cancer cell does, without regard for the overall requirement of the host. The

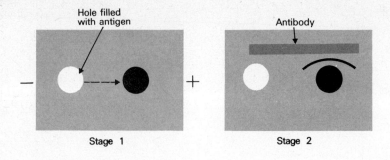

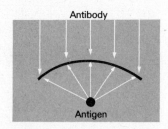

FIGURE 2.8. The principle of immunoelectrophoresis. *Stage 1 :* Electrophoresis of antigen in agar gel. Antigen moves to hypothetical position shown. *Stage 2 :* Current stopped. Trough cut in agar and filled with antibody. Pecipitin arc formed.

Because antigen theoretically at a point source diffuses radially and antibody from the trough diffuses with a plane front, they meet in optimal proportions for precipitation along an arc. The arc is closest to the trough at the point where antigen is in highest concentration.

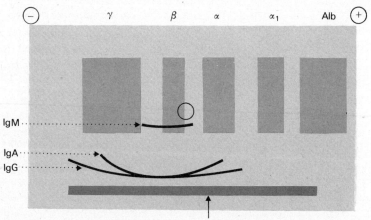

FIGURE 2.9. Major human immunoglobulin classes demonstrated by immunoelectrophoretic analysis of human serum using a rabbit antiserum in the trough. The position of the main electrophoretic fractions of serum are indicated. Three of the five major immunoglobulin classes can be recognized: immunoglobulin G (IgG), immunoglobulin A (IgA) and immunoglobulin M (IgM). The IgG precipitin arc extends from the γ region well into the α_2-globulin mobility range.

patient then possesses enormous numbers of identical cells derived as a clone from the original cell and they all synthesize the same immunoglobulin—the myeloma or M-protein—which appears in the serum, sometimes in very high concentrations. By purification of the myeloma protein we can obtain a preparation of an immunoglobulin having a unique structure. These myeloma proteins have been studied in two ways: amino acid analysis and the recognition of major characteristic groups on the molecules using specific antibodies produced in experimental animals.

STRUCTURAL VARIATION IN RELATION TO ANTIBODY SPECIFICITY

Amino acid analysis of a number of purified myeloma proteins has revealed that, within a given major immunoglobulin class

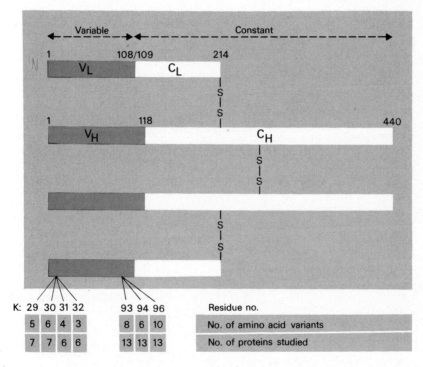

FIGURE 2.10. Showing the regions of IgG with relatively variable (▬) and constant (▭) amino acid composition. The terms 'V region' and 'C region' are used to designate the variable and constant regions respectively. 'V_L' and 'C_L' are generic terms for these regions on the light chain and 'V_H' and 'C_H' specify variable and constant regions on the heavy chain. The amino acid residues are numbered starting from the N-terminal end. C_L starts at residue 108 for κ-types and 109 for λ (see also figure 4.6).

such as IgG, the N-terminal portions of both heavy and light chains show quite considerable variations whereas the remaining parts of the chains are relatively constant in structure (figure 2.10). Within the variable region, a number of amino acid positions in the peptide chains are substituted by a variety of amino acids and certain residues exhibit a notable *hypervariability* (e.g. figure 2.10). The most attractive view, supported by the latest X-ray analysis, is that these 'hot spots', three on the light and three on the heavy chain, lie relatively close to each other to form the antigen binding site (figure 2.11), their heterogeneity ensuring diversity in combining specificities

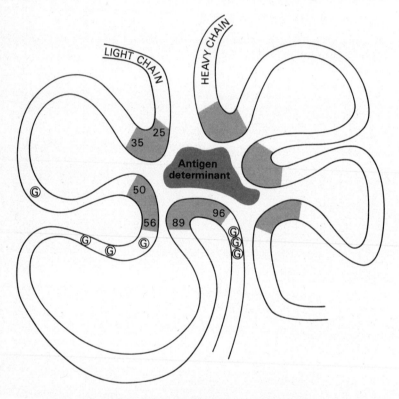

FIGURE 2.11. Formation of an antigen binding site by spatial apposition of hypervariable regions (hot spots: ▬) on light and heavy chains. Numbers refer to amino acid residues. Glycine residues (Ⓖ) are invariably present at the positions indicated whatever the specificity or animal species of the immunoglobulin and Wu and Kabat have suggested that the flexibility of bond angle in this amino acid is essential for the effective formation of a binding site. A theoretical model of a light chain constructed on the assumption that the bond angle between a given amino acid and its nearest neighbours will be similar to that found on X-ray analysis of the same tripeptide in other proteins is consistent with the idea that the 'hot spots' form one side of a cleft (Kabat & Wu).

through variation in the shape and nature of the surface they create (cf. p. 14).

That these variable regions on heavy and light chains both contribute to antibody specificity is suggested by experiments in which isolated chains were examined for their antigen combining power. In general, varying degrees of residual activity were associated with the heavy chains but relatively little, if any, with the light chains (although light chain dimers were recently shown to be more effective); on recombination, however, there was always a significant increase in antigen-binding capacity.

More direct attempts to identify the amino acid residues associated with the combining site have been made by Singer and others using a technique called 'affinity-labelling'. In this, a hapten is equipped with a chemically reactive side chain which will form covalent links with adjacent amino acids after combination of the hapten with antibody, so labelling residues in the neighbourhood of the combining site. A modification introduced by Porter and his colleagues utilizes a 'flick-knife' principle. The hapten with an azide side chain combines with its antibody and is then illuminated with ultraviolet light; this converts the azide to the reactive nitrene radical which will covalently link to almost any organic group with which it comes in contact (e.g. figure 2.12). Preliminary results indicate that the affinity label binds to both heavy and light chains in the hypervariable regions. This technique should help to define the amino acid residues which go to make up the combining site. There is no doubt that the electron microscopic studies with divalent hapten (cf. figures 2.6 and 2.7) show the antigen-combining sites to be associated with the N-terminal region of the molecule which at least bears out the overall view that the variable regions are implicated in antibody specificity.

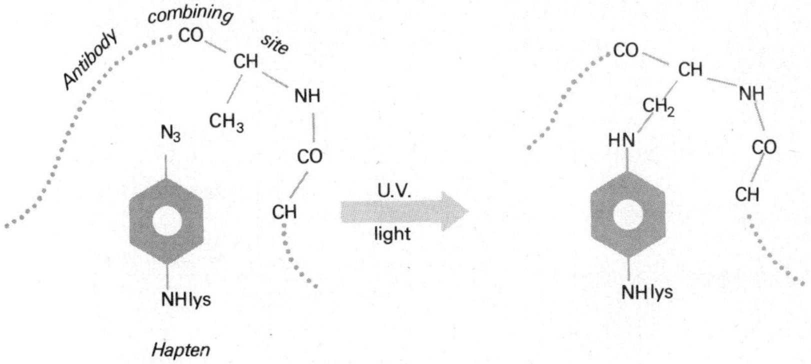

FIGURE 2.12. Affinity labelling: The hapten binds to its antibody and the azide group activated by ultraviolet light loses N_2 and the resulting radical combines with an adjacent amino acid—in this hypothetical example an alanine residue. Analysis of the protein after digestion would show the alanine to be labelled with the hapten and implicate this residue in the combining site. Studies by Fleet G.W.J., Porter R.R. & Knowles J.R. (*Nature* 1969, **224**, 511) indicate that the affinity label combines with heavy and light chains in a ratio of approximately 3·5:1.

Even the 'constant' portions of the immunoglobulin peptide chains which are not directly concerned in antigen binding show considerable heterogeneity. This has largely been analysed through the recognition of characteristic groupings on the molecules by use of specific antisera raised usually in other species. Let us consider, for example, studies on human immunoglobulin light chains.

Light chains

A convenient source of human material is the urinary Bence–Jones' protein which is found in a proportion of patients with myeloma. The Bence–Jones' protein represents a dimer of light chains derived from the pool used in the synthesis of the myeloma protein. By raising antisera in rabbits to a number of Bence–Jones' proteins it was found that light chains could be divided into two groups (called *kappa* (κ) and *lambda* (λ)) depending upon their reactions with the antisera. The Bence–Jones' light chains of the κ-group all gave precipitin reactions with anti-κ sera but no reaction with anti-λ sera. Parallel reactions were always obtained with the parent myeloma protein as would be expected if they were derived from light chains produced by one clone of myeloma plasma cells (figure 2.13).

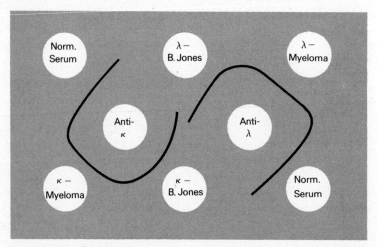

FIGURE 2.13. Precipitation reactions in agar-gel using antisera prepared against κ and λ Bence–Jones' proteins (urinary light chain dimers). The anti-κ reacted with κ but not λ light chains and gave reactions of 'identity' with the related myeloma protein and with normal serum. Parallel results were obtained with the anti-λ serum.

The reactions with normal serum show that molecules with κ- and λ-chains are present. They occur on different molecules and approximately 65 per cent of the immunoglobulin molecules in normal serum are of κ-type, the remainder being λ-type. It is of interest that myeloma proteins of type κ occur with nearly twice the frequency of type λ, suggesting that cells synthesizing molecules with λ-chains carry the same risk of becoming malignant as those making κ-chains. The $\kappa : \lambda$ ratio varies in different species.

Heavy chains

Similar studies using antisera prepared against normal and myeloma proteins have established the existence of *five* major types of heavy chain in the human, each of which gives rise to a distinct immunoglobulin class. As mentioned earlier these are IgG, IgA, IgM, IgD and IgE (alternative abbreviations not now accepted are γG, γA, γM, γD and γE, which epitomized a persistent dedication to the historical but incorrect view that all antibodies are of γ-globulin mobility). But whereas each immunoglobulin class is associated with a particular type of heavy chain, they all have κ- and λ-light chains; thus each myeloma protein so far studied, whatever its class, has possessed light chains of either κ- or λ-specificity (but never of both together).

We have already considered the view that the variable portion of the immunoglobulin molecule is bound up with antibody specificity and all classes have been shown to have binding affinity for antigen associated with the Fab regions. What of the constant region, particularly the Fc part of the heavy chain backbone which makes no contribution to specificity? Almost certainly the Fc structure directs the *biological activity* of the antibody molecule. As will be seen below, it determines to some extent the distribution of the immunoglobulin throughout the body, e.g. the selective passage of IgG across the placenta and perhaps the secretion of IgA into the external body fluids. But also, after combination with antigen a new or enhanced activity such as the ability to fix complement, or to bind effectively to macrophages or to cause mast cell degranulation may arise. Whether this occurs through an allosteric change in Fc conformation due to the opening of the 'hinge' or through the increased binding due to the multivalent Fc sites present in an immune complex (cf. bonus effect of multivalency p. 15), or both, is unresolved. Each of these functions may require a different type of Fc structure and hence

33

amino acid sequence. Thus the multiplicity of Fc structures as expressed in the different immunoglobulin classes (and *sub-classes vide infra*) may be looked upon as a system which has evolved to provide antibodies with different biological capabilities in relation to antigens.

In summary, the variable part provides specificity for binding antigen; the constant part is associated with different biological properties which vary from one immunoglobulin class to another, depending upon the primary structure, and which may require combination with antigen for their activation.

Immunoglobulin domains

In addition to the *interchain* disulphide bonds which bridge heavy and light chains, each immunoglobulin peptide chain has internal disulphide links. These *intrachain* disulphide bonds form loops in the peptide chain as shown in figure 2.14 and

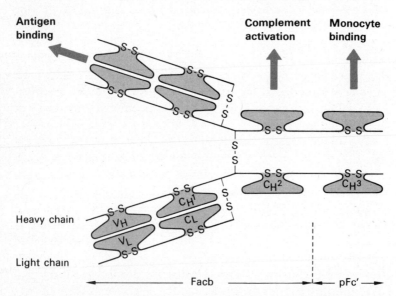

FIGURE 2.14. Immunoglobulin domains. Each loop in the peptide chain formed by an *intrachain* disulphide bond represents a single domain (shaded) and these are labelled V_H, C_{H1} etc. as indicated. The domains in the constant parts of the light and heavy chains are marked with a cross and show homology (i.e. similarities in amino acid structure). Each domain appears to be specialized for a specific function as shown. The involvement of the C_{H2} region in complement activation is indicated by the activity of the plasmin Facb fragment which contains the C_{H2} domain, and the inactivity of the F(ab')$_2$ fragment which lacks it. The pepsin pFc' fragment which bears the C_{H3} domain can bind directly to the monocyte surface and inhibit the formation of Fc rosettes with antibody coated red cells.

34

Edelman has suggested that each of the loops is compactly folded to form a globular domain and further that each domain subserves a separate function.

Thus the variable region domains (V_L and V_H) are responsible for the formation of a specific antigen-binding site. The C_{H2} region binds C1q to initiate the classical complement sequence (cf. p. 121) while adherence to the monocyte surface is mediated through the terminal C_{H3} domain (figure 2.14).

Comparison of immunoglobulin classes

The physical and biological characteristics of the five major immunoglobulin classes in the human are summarized in tables 2.1 and 2.2. The following comments are intended to supplement this information.

TABLE 2.1. Physical properties of major human immunoglobulin classes

WHO Designation	IgG	IgA	IgM	IgD	IgE
Sedimentation coefficient	$7S$	$7S$, $9S$, $11S^*$	$19S$	$7S$	$8S$
Molecular weight	150,000	160,000 and polymers	900,000	185,000	200,000
Number of basic 4-peptide units	1	1, 2*	5	1	1
Heavy chains	γ	α	μ	δ	ε
Light chains $\kappa + \lambda$	$\kappa + \lambda$	$\kappa + \lambda$	$\kappa + \lambda$	$\kappa + \lambda$	$\kappa + \lambda$
Molecular formula†	$\gamma_2\kappa_2 \cdot \gamma_2\lambda_2$	$(\alpha_2\kappa_2)_{1-3}$ $(\alpha_2\lambda_2)_{1-3}$ $(\alpha_2\kappa_2)_2 S^*$ $(\alpha_2\lambda_2)_2 S^*$	$(\mu_2\kappa_2)_5$ $(\mu_2\lambda_2)_5$	$\delta_2\kappa_2(\delta_2\lambda_2?)$	$\varepsilon_2\kappa_2 \cdot \varepsilon_2\lambda_2$
Valency for antigen binding	2	2, (? polymers)	5(10)	?	2
Concentration range in normal serum	8–16 mg/ml	1·4–4 mg/ml	0·5–2 mg/ml	0–0·4 mg/ml	17–450 ng/ml‡
% total immunoglobulin	80	13	6	1	0·002
Carbohydrate content, %	3	8	12	13	12

* Dimer in external secretions carries secretory component—S.
† IgA polymers and IgM contain J chain.
‡ ng = 10^{-9} g.

	IgG	IgA	IgM	IgD	IgE
Major characteristics	Most abundant Ig of internal body fluids particularly extra-vascular where combats micro-organisms and their toxins	Major Ig in sero-mucous secretions where it defends external body surfaces	Very effective agglutinator; produced early in immune response—effective first line defence vs. bacteraemia	Present on lymphocyte surface of newborn	Raised in parasitic infections Responsible for symptoms of atopic allergy
Complement fixation	+	−	+	?	−
Cross placenta	+	−	−	−	−
Fix to mast cells (in homologous skin) and basophils	−	−	−	−	+
Cytophilic binding to macrophages	+	−	−	−	−

Immunoglobulin G

During the secondary response IgG is probably the major immunoglobulin to be synthesized. Through its ability to cross the placenta it provides a major line of defence against infection for the first few weeks of a baby's life which may be further reinforced by the transfer of colostral IgG across the gut mucosa in the neonate. IgG diffuses more readily than the other immunoglobulins into the extravascular body spaces where as the predominant species it carries the major burden of neutralizing bacterial toxins and of binding to micro-organisms to enhance their phagocytosis. The complexes of bacteria with IgG antibody can adhere to phagocytic cells because these cells have specialized surface receptors for sites on the Fc portion of IgG (and also of C3). Other cells display surface receptors capable of binding to the Fc regions of IgG; thus red cells coated with IgG antibodies will adhere to B-lymphocytes (cf. p. 56) to form rosettes. Furthermore, only IgG antibodies coating target cells will sensitize them for extracellular killing by K-cells (cf. 129). Although unable to bind firmly to mast cells in human skin, IgG alone among the human immunoglobulins has the somewhat useless property of fixing to guinea pig skin. The thesis that the biological individuality of different immunoglobulin classes is dependent on the heavy chain constant regions, particularly the Fc, is amply borne out in relationship to the activities we have discussed such as transplacental passage, complement fixation and binding to various cell types, where function has been shown to be mediated by the Fc part of the molecule.

With respect to overall regulation of IgG levels in the body, the catabolic rate appears to depend directly upon the total IgG concentration whereas synthesis is entirely governed by antigen stimulation so that in germ-free animals, for example, IgG levels are extremely low but rise rapidly on transfer to a normal environment.

Immunoglobulin A

This is present in serum mainly as the 7S monomer but tends to form polymers spontaneously through association with a cysteine-rich polypeptide called J-chain. IgA appears selectively in the sero-mucous secretions such as saliva, tears, nasal fluids, sweat, colostrum and secretions of the lung and gastro-intestinal tract where it clearly has the job of defending the exposed external surfaces of the body against attack by micro-organisms. It appears in these fluids essentially as the dimer stabilized against proteolysis by combination with another protein—the secretory component which is synthesized by local epithelial cells and has a single peptide chain of molecular weight 60,000. The IgA is synthesized locally by plasma cells and released as a dimer. If dimerization occurred randomly *after* release, dimers of mixed specificity would be formed which would not be as effective in combining with antigen as those of single specificity which would have a higher valency. IgA antibodies may function by inhibiting the adherence of coated micro-organisms to the surface of mucosal cells thereby preventing entry into the body tissues. There are also interesting reports of a synergism between IgA, lysozyme and complement in the killing of certain coliform organisms, and of the ability of aggregated IgA to bind polymorphs and to activate the C3 bypass (p. 122) rather than the classical complement pathway.

Immunoglobulin M

Often referred to as the macroglobulin antibodies because of their high molecular weight, IgM molecules are polymers of five 4-peptide subunits each bearing an extra C_H domain. As with IgA, polymerisation of the subunits depends upon the presence of J-chain(s) and the structure as at present envisaged by Hilschman is illustrated in figure 2.15a. Under negative

37

staining in the electron-microscope, the free molecule assumes a 'star' shape but when combined as an antibody with an antigenic surface membrane it can adopt a 'crab-like' configuration (figures 2.15b and c). The theoretical combining valency is of course 10 but this is only observed on interaction with small haptens; with larger antigens the effective valency falls to 5 and this must be attributed to some form of steric restriction.

Because of their high valency, IgM antibodies are extremely

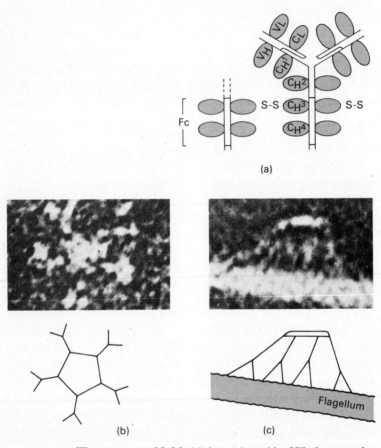

(a)

(b)   (c)

FIGURE 2.15. The structure of IgM: (a) As envisaged by Hilschman and colleagues showing the extra (C_{H4}) domain and the disulphide linkage between C_{H3} domains which enable the pentamer to be formed (b) As shown by electron microscopy of a human Waldenström's macroglobulin in free solution adopting a 'star'-shaped configuration (c) As revealed in an E.M. preparation of specific sheep IgM antibody bound to *Salmonella paratyphi* flagellum where the immunoglobulin has assumed a 'crab-like' conformation in establishing its links with antigen. (Electron micrographs—kindly provided by Dr. A. Feinstein and Dr. E.A. Munn—are negatively stained preparations of magnification 2,000,000 ×, i.e. 1 mm respresents 5 Å.)

efficient agglutinating and cytolytic agents and since they appear early in the response to infection and are largely confined to the blood stream, it is likely that they play a role of particular importance in cases of bacteraemia. The isohaemagglutinins (anti-A, anti-B) and many of the 'natural' antibodies to microorganisms are usually IgM; antibodies to the typhoid 'O' antigen (endotoxin) and the 'WR' antibodies in syphilis also tend to be found in this class. IgM would appear to precede IgG in the phylogeny of the immune response in vertebrates.

Immunoglobulin D

This class was recognized through the discovery of a myeloma protein which did not have the antigenic specificity of IgG, A or M, although it reacted with antibodies to immunoglobulin light chains and had the basic four-peptide structure. Until recently, no antibody activity had been unequivocally demonstrated in IgD but there are now reports of IgD antinuclear antibodies and of antibodies to BSA in gut fluids. An exciting development has been the demonstration of IgD on the surface of a proportion of cord blood lymphocytes and it is tempting to regard this as an early receptor which later gives way to IgM and other immunoglobulins as the cell differentiates further (Rowe).

Immunoglobulin E

Only very low concentrations of IgE are present in serum and only a very small proportion of the plasma cells in the body are synthesizing this immunoglobulin. It is not surprising, therefore, that so far only two cases of IgE myeloma have been recognized compared with tens of thousands of IgG paraproteinaemias. IgE antibodies remain firmly fixed for an extended period when injected into human skin where they are probably bound to mast cells. Contact with antigen leads to degranulation of the mast cells with release of vasoactive amines. This process is responsible for the symptoms of hayfever and of extrinsic asthma when patients with atopic allergy come in contact with the allergen, e.g. grass pollen. The main *physiological* role of IgE is still uncertain but it has been noticed that the serum level rises considerably on infection with certain parasites particularly helminths; it is thought that histamine release resulting from contact of parasite antigens with mast-cell bound IgE antibody in the gut wall facilitates ejection of the intruders.

TABLE 2.3. Comparison of human IgG subclasses

	IgG1	IgG2	IgG3	IgG4
% of total IgG in normal serum	65	23	8	4
Electrophoretic mobility	slow	slow	slow	fast
Spontaneous aggregation	−	−	+++	−
Gm allotypes	a,y,f,x	n	b,b_3,b_4,s, t,c,g	
Ga site reacting with rheumatoid factor*	+++	+++	−	+++
Combination with staphylococcal A protein	+++	+++	−	+++
Cross placenta	++	±	++	++
Complement fixation (C1 pathway)	+++	++	++++	±
Binding to monocytes	+++	+	+++	±
Binding to heterologous skin	++	−	++	++
Blocking IgE binding	−	−	−	+
Antibody dominance	Anti-Rh	Anti-dextran Anti-levan	Anti-Rh	Anti Factor VIII

* Other rheumatoid factors apparently react with Gm specific sites.

IMMUNOGLOBULIN SUBCLASSES

Antigenic analysis of IgG myelomas revealed further variation and showed that they could be grouped into four *subclasses* now termed IgG1, IgG2, IgG3 and IgG4. The differences all lie in the heavy chains which have been labelled γ1, γ2, γ3 and γ4 respectively. These heavy chains show considerable homology and have certain structures in common with each other—the ones which react with specific anti-IgG antisera—but each has one or more additional structures characteristic of its own subclass arising from differences in primary amino acid composition and in disulphide bridging. These give rise to differences in biological behaviour which are only now becoming apparent (table 2.3).

Two subclasses of IgA have also been found. The IgA2 subclass is unusual in that it lacks interchain disulphide bonds between heavy and light chains. Class and subclass variation is not restricted to human immunoglobulins but is a feature of all the higher mammals so far studied; monkey, sheep, rabbit, guinea-pig, rat and mouse.

OTHER IMMUNOGLOBULIN VARIANTS

Aside from the structural heterogeneity in the heavy chains associated with class and subclass specificity, further *isotypic* subvariants, all present in the serum of normal subjects, have been identified (table 2.4). *Allotypes* represent yet a further type of variation within a given subclass which depends upon the existence of allelic forms. In somewhat the same way as the red cells in genetically different individuals can differ in terms of the blood group antigen system A, B, O, so the Ig heavy chains differ in the expression of their allotypic groups. This usually involves one or two amino acids in the peptide chain. Take for example the Gma locus on IgG1 (table 2.3). An individual classed as Gma+ would show this group on each of his IgG1 molecules and this corresponds with the peptide sequence: Asp.Glu.Leu.Thr.Lys. Another person whose IgG1 molecules were Gma− would have the sequence Met.Glu.Glu.Thr.Lys, i.e. two amino acids different. These groups are recognizable by the use of appropriate anti-γ-globulin antibodies present in the sera of patients with rheumatoid arthritis. To date, 25 genetic markers (Gm groups) have been found on the heavy chain and a further three (the Inv groups) on the light chain.

Allotypic markers have also been found on the immunoglobulins of rabbits and of mice using reagents prepared by immunizing one animal with an immune complex obtained with antibodies from another animal of the same species. In some instances *idiotypic* antibodies were obtained when donor and recipient animal were of the same allotypes; here the specificity was directed only against the particular antibody in the donor serum which had been used for forming the immunizing immune complex. Although the existence of idiotypic determinants on purified antibodies has come to light only recently, it has long been known that antibodies to a given human myeloma protein raised in rabbits recognize a configuration unique to that myeloma after the antiserum has been absorbed with normal human serum (although that idiotype would be present on a few of the immunoglobulin molecules in normal serum the number would be insufficient to neutralize the anti-idiotype antibodies). The idiotype determinants are located in the variable part of the antibody either in the combining site or in regions determining the configuration of the site. Thus in a number of cases the reaction of an anti-idiotypic serum directed against an anti-hapten antibody can be inhibited by prior addition of hapten. The existence of anti-idiotypes provides further support

TABLE 2.4. Summary of immunoglobulin variants

Type of variation	Distribution	Variant	Location	Examples
ISOTYPIC	All variants present in serum of a normal individual	Classes	C_H	IgM, IgE
		Subclasses	C_H	IgA1, IgA2
		Types	C_L	κ, λ
		Subtypes	C_L	λOz^+, λOz^-
		Subgroups	V_L	$V_{\kappa I}$, $V_{\kappa II}$, $V_{\kappa III}$
ALLOTYPIC	Allelic forms: not present in all individuals	Allotypes	Mainly C_H/C_L sometimes V_H/V_L	Gm groups (human) b_4, b_5, b_6, b_9 (rabbit light chains)
IDIOTYPIC	Individually specific to each immuno-globulin molecule	Idiotypes	Variable regions	Determinant identified by antibody specific to an *individual* myeloma protein or antibody molecule

for the idea that each antibody has a unique structure. These antisera may provide useful reagents, e.g. for identification of specific immune complexes in patients' sera, for recognition of V_L type amyloid in subjects excreting Bence-Jones proteins, for detection of residual monoclonal protein after therapy and perhaps for selecting lymphocytes with certain surface receptors.

Further reading

Dubiski S. (1972) Genetics & regulation of immunoglobulin allotypes. *Med.Clinics Nth.America*, **56**, 557.

Edelman G.M. *et al.* (1969) Complete sequence of human IgG1. *Proc.Nat. Acad.Sci.*, **63**, 78.

Kabat E.A. & Wu T.T. (1972) Construction of a 3-dimensional model of the polypeptide backbone of the variable region of the κ immunoglobulin light chains. *Proc.Nat.Acad.Sci.*, **69**, 960.

Leslie R.G.Q. & Cohen S. (1973) The active sites of immunoglobulin molecules. In *Essays in Fundamental Immunology 1*, page 1. Blackwell Scientific Publications, Oxford.

Milstein C. & Pink J.R.L. (1970) Structure and evolution of immunoglobulins. *Progr.Biophys.Mol.Biol.*, **21**, 211.

Natvig J.B. & Kunkel H. (1973) Human immunoglobulins: classes, subclasses, genetic variants and idiotypes. *Adv. in Immunology*, **16**, 1.

Poljak R.J. *et al.* (1973) Three-dimensional structure of the Fab' fragment of a human immunoglobulin at 2·8-Å resolution. *Proc.Nat.Acad.Sci.*, **70**, 3305.

3 The synthesis of antibody

Two types of immune response

When antigen enters the body, two different types of immuno-logical reaction may occur:

1. The synthesis and release of free antibody into the blood and other body fluids (*humoral antibody*). This antibody acts, for example, by direct combination with and neutralization of bacterial toxins, by coating bacteria to enhance their phago-cytosis and so on.
2. The production of 'sensitized' lymphocytes which have antibody-like molecules on their surface ('cell-bound anti-body'). These are the effectors of *cell-mediated immunity* expressed in such reactions as the rejection of skin transplants and the 'delayed' hypersensitivity to tuberculin (Mantoux test) seen in individuals immune to tubercle infection.

Role of the small lymphocyte

The central importance of the lymphocyte for both types of immune response was established largely by the work of Gowans. By labelling the lymphocytes with radioisotope and following their fate in the body it could be shown that there is a pool of recirculating lymphocytes which pass from the blood into the lymph nodes, spleen and other tissues and back to the blood by the major lymphatic channels such as the thoracic duct.

PRIMARY RESPONSE

When rats are depleted of their lymphocytes by chronic drainage of lymph from the thoracic duct by an indwelling cannula, they have a grossly impaired ability to mount a primary antibody response to antigens such as tetanus toxoid and sheep red blood cells, or to reject a skin graft. Immunological reactivity can be restored by injecting thoracic duct lymphocytes obtained from another rat. The same effect can be obtained if the thoracic duct cells are first incubated at $37°C$ for 24 hours before injection: this treatment kills off large and medium sized cells and leaves only the small lymphocytes. Thus the small lymphocyte is necessary for the primary response to antigen.

Transfer experiments have also shown that small lymphocytes can become antibody synthesizing cells (plasma cells) and effector cells in transplantation reactions (probably lymphoblasts).

SECONDARY RESPONSE—MEMORY

An immunologically 'virgin' rat, i.e. one which has had no previous contact with a specific antigen, may be inoculated with small lymphocytes from a rat which has already given a primary response to that antigen. Challenge of the recipient rat with antigen leads to a secondary type response with the rapid production of high-titre antibodies. If the recipient had not been injected with small lymphocytes from the 'primed' donor, a primary response with the relatively slow development of lower titre antibodies would have been seen (figure 3.1). Thus the small lymphocytes carry the *memory* of the first contact with antigen.

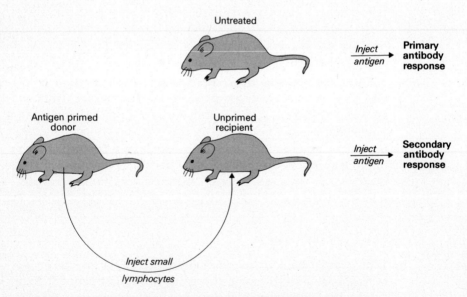

FIGURE 3.1. Transfer of immunological memory by small lymphocytes from primed donor rat. In these transfer experiments, genetically identical animals of the same strain are used to prevent complications arising from transplantation reactions between the transferred lymphocytes and the host.

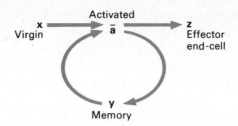

FIGURE 3.2. Possible relationship between x, y and z lymphocytic cells (developed from Sercarz and Coons). Most, if not all stages are antigen-driven. Proliferation must occur at some stage between x and y (since there is an expanded pool of antigen-sensitive memory cells after a primary response) and between y and z (since e.g. antibody-forming cells in mitosis have been observed).

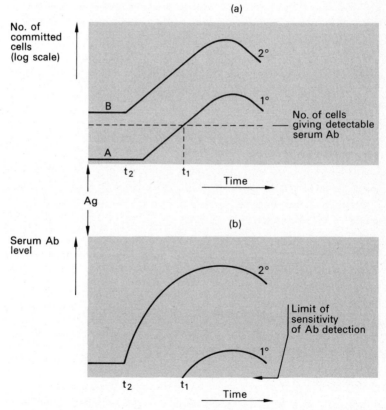

FIGURE 3.3. Kinetics of (a) the cellular and (b) the corresponding serum antibody changes during the primary and secondary responses to antigen. The interval between antigen challenge and proliferation in the primary (A) is probably greater than the corresponding period for the secondary response (B) and some further time must elapse before the population of Ab-forming cells is large enough to give detectable antibody (however, the more sensitive the detection method used, the shorter this time must be).

45

We may recognize at least three cell types representing different phases in the differentiation of the immunocompetent cell: (x) virgin lymphocytes which have not yet experienced the ecstasy of contact with antigen, (y) memory cells and (z) antibody-forming cells derived from x cells as a result of antigenic stimulation. One possible relationship which postulates a common activated blast cell intermediate is suggested in figure 3.2.

In the primary response, a relatively small number of x cells specific for the antigen are induced to differentiate and proliferate but some time (t_1 in figure 3.3) must elapse before the number of antibody-forming cells has been expanded sufficiently to produce detectable serum antibody. By contrast, in the secondary response the animal starts with an expanded population of y cells whose proliferative response to antigen is more immediately reflected by an increase in serum antibody which reaches a high level relative to the primary response because of the greater number of committed cells produced (figure 3.3a and b). The net result is the more rapid, more intense response characteristically associated with the second contact with antigen (cf. figure 1.2).

The thymus

This gland is made up essentially of epithelial cells and large numbers of lymphocytes, many of them dividing. The occurrence of frequent thymic abnormalities in children with immunological deficiency disorders led to the suggestion that the thymus was related in some way to the development of immune responses (Good and colleagues). The relationship was clarified by Miller's demonstration that removal of the thymus gland in mice at birth led to:

(i) decrease in circulating lymphocytes;

(ii) severe impairment of graft rejection;

(iii) reduced humoral antibody response to some but not all antigens;

(iv) wasting after 1–3 months—probably a result of inability to combat infection effectively since neonatally thymectomized mice reared under germ-free conditions did not waste.

The defects caused by neonatal thymectomy can be partially reversed by soluble thymus extracts and there is increasing evidence for a hormone, 'thymosin'.

X-irradiation of adult mice destroys the ability of their lymphocytes to divide and hence their immunological respon-

46

siveness. This can be restored by injection of bone marrow cells. However bone marrow cells fail to restore X-irradiated adult mice which have been thymectomized; on the other hand, adult spleen and lymph node cells were effective. It is thus concluded that the thymus acts on primitive cells coming from the bone marrow to make them immunologically competent.

The Bursa of Fabricius

In chickens, another lymphoid organ termed the Bursa of Fabricius can be recognized. It is similar to the thymus and also embryologically derived from gut epithelium. Just as the thymus appears to act as a central lymphoid organ controlling the maturation of lymphocytes concerned largely with cell-mediated immunity, so the Bursa of Fabricius is responsible for the development of immunocompetence in cells destined to make humoral antibody. This differentiation of function may be readily seen from the results of the experiments documented in table 3.1: the thymus or bursa was removed from newborn chicks which were then irradiated to inactivate any competent lymphocytes which had already reached the peripheral tissues. After several weeks the chickens were tested and it was found that bursectomy had a profound effect on humoral antibody synthesis but did not unduly influence the cell mediated reactions responsible for tuberculin hypersensitivity and graft rejection. On the other hand, as in the mice, thymectomy grossly impaired cell-mediated reactions and had some effect on antibody production.

TABLE 3.1. Effect of neonatal bursectomy and thymectomy on the development of immunological competence in the chicken (From Cooper M.D., Peterson R.D.A., South M.A. & Good R.A., *J.exp.Med.* 1966, **123**, 75, with permission of the editors)

All X-irradiated after birth	Peripheral blood lymphocyte count	Ig concn.	Antibody	Delayed hypersensitivity to tuberculin	Graft rejection
Intact	14,800	+ +	+ + +	+ +	+ +
Thymectom-ized	9,000	+ +	+	−	−
Bursectomized	13,200	−	−	+	+

Two populations of lymphocytes: T- and B-cells

There thus appear to be two different small lymphocyte populations:

(i) *T-lymphocytes*, processed by or in some way dependent on the thymus, and responsible for cell-mediated immunity;

(ii) *B-lymphocytes*, bursa-dependent, and concerned in the synthesis of circulating antibody.

Both populations on appropriate stimulation by antigen proliferate and undergo morphological changes (figure 3.4). The B-lymphocytes develop into the plasma cell series. The mature plasma cell (figure 3.5b) is actively synthesizing and secreting antibody and has a well-developed rough surfaced endoplasmic reticulum (figure 3.5f) characteristic of a cell producing protein for 'export'. T-lymphocytes transform to

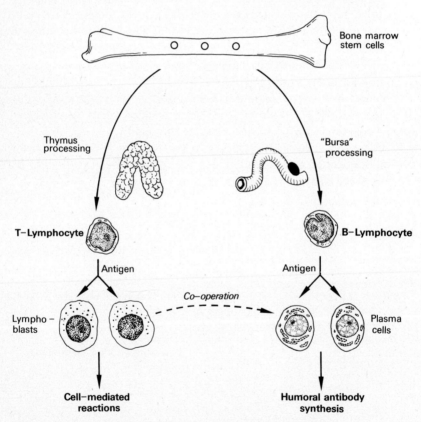

FIGURE 3.4. Processing of bone marrow cells by thymus and gut-associated central lymphoid tissue to become immunocompetent T- and B-lymphocytes respectively. Proliferation and transformation to cells of the lymphoblast and plasma cell series occurs on antigenic stimulation.

48

lymphoblasts (figure 3.5i) which in the electron microscope are seen to have virtually no rough-surfaced endoplasmic reticulum although there are abundant free ribosomes, either single or as polysomes (figure 3.5j). These cells are concerned with the synthesis of their own components but do not secrete appreciable amounts of free antibody. Their high ribosome content makes them basophilic so that they show superficial resemblance to plasmablasts in the light microscope. However, no antibody can be detected in their cytoplasm using immunofluorescent methods.

The equivalent of the bursa in man and other mammals has not yet been clearly defined although gut-associated lymphoid tissue such as the tonsil, appendix, Peyer's patches, lymphoid follicles themselves and haemopoietic tissue have been nominated as possible candidates. Nonetheless there is considerable circumstantial evidence indicating morphological compartmentation of the two major types of immune response. Certain regions in peripheral lymphoid tissue, around the splenic arterioles and in the paracortical areas of the lymph nodes, show severe lymphocyte depletion after neonatal thymectomy, whereas the lymphoid follicles are unaffected. Comparable abnormalities are found in hairless mice (the so-called 'nude' mice homozygous for the *nu* gene) which are born with gross thymic dysplasia. When a cell-mediated immunological response is elicited in a normal animal, say by a skin graft or by painting chemicals such as picryl chloride on the skin to induce contact hypersensitivity, there is a marked proliferation of cells in the thymus-dependent area of the lymph node and typical lymphoblasts are seen (figure 3.6). On the other hand, stimulation of antibody formation by the 'thymus independent' antigen pneumococcus polysaccharide leads to proliferation in the cortical lymphoid follicles with development of germinal centres and the migration of plasma cells to the medullary cords; the thymus-dependent paracortical region remains inactive and no cellular hypersensitivity to the polysaccharide can be detected.

Other evidence stems from selective immunological deficiencies in man (see chapter 7). Defective cellular immunity is associated with depletion of thymus-dependent areas in the lymphoid tissue while cases with immunoglobulin deficiency show poor development of follicular structures.

IDENTIFICATION OF B- AND T-LYMPHOCYTES

From the morphological standpoint there is little to choose between B- and T- small lymphocytes examined by conventional light or electron microscopy but a startling difference has

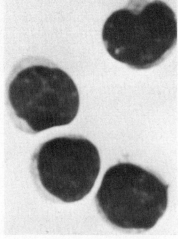
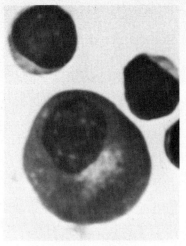

(a) Small lymphocyte ×2800   (b) Plasma cell ×2800

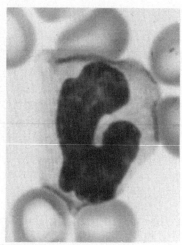
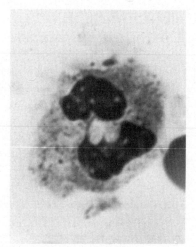

(c) Monocyte ×2800   (d) Polymorph ×2800

FIGURE 3.5. Morphology of cells connected with immune responses.
(a) Small lymphocyte, × 2,800   (b) Plasma cell, × 2,800
(c) Monocyte, × 2,800   (d) Polymorph, × 2,800
(e) Small lymphocyte, × 13,000   (f) Plasma cell, × 10,000
(g) Monocyte, × 10,000   (h) Polymorph, × 10,000
(i) Transformed lymphocyte (lymphoblast), × 2,800.
(j) Transformed lymphocyte (lymphoblast), × 7,000.
(Courtesy of Miss V. Petts)

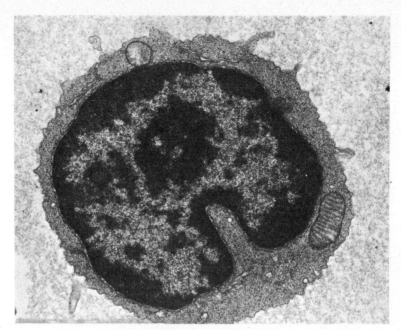

(e) Small lymphocyte ×13000

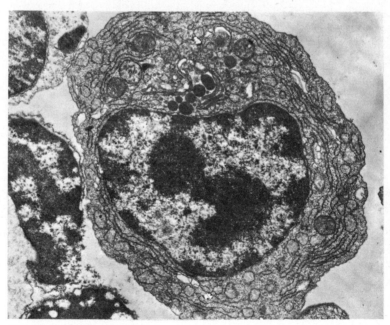

(f) Plasma cell ×10000

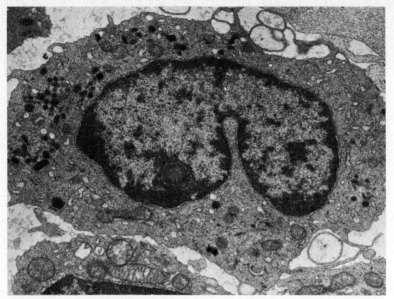

(g) Monocyte ×10000

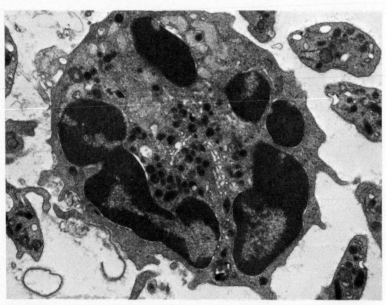

(h) Polymorph ×10000

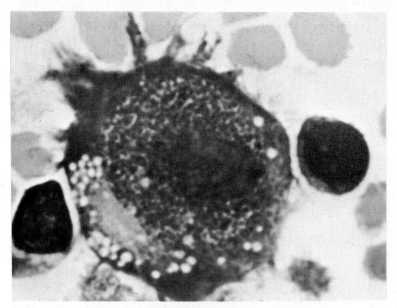

(i) Transformed lymphocyte (lymphoblast) ×2800

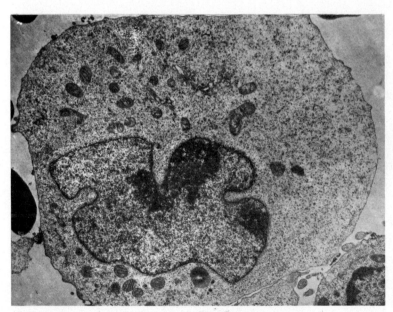

(j) Transformed lymphocyte (lymphoblast) ×7000

53

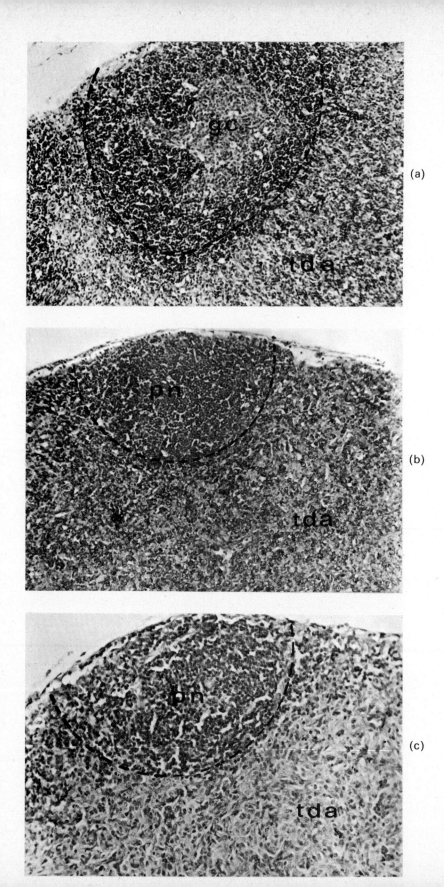

(a)

(b)

(c)

TABLE 3.2. Tests for surface markers on B and T cells

Lymphocytes	Immunofluorescent staining for:		Rosette (cluster) formation with:			Approx. % of human blood lymphocytes
	Ig	Sp. Ag shared with brain	sheep r.b.c. alone	Fc coated r.b.c.	C3 coated r.b.c.	
T	−	+ +	+ +*	+†	+	70
B	+ +	−	−	+ +	+ +	25

* Human T-cells.   † Activated T-cells.

been picked up by the scanning electron-microscope; T-cells present a bland flat surface whereas B-lymphocytes have rather an agitated appearance with numerous surface projections. However this instrument is not exactly everyone's plaything and most ordinary mortals have exploited a variety of surface markers to differentiate the two populations of cells (table 3.2).

Immunoglobulins are readily demonstrable on the surface of B- but not T-lymphocytes using an immunofluorescent technique with reagents such as fluorescein-labelled anti-immuno-globulin light chain (cf. figure 3.8a). It appears that a large proportion of B-cells bear surface IgM, probably as monomer, but many stain with antisera directed against the Fc portion of other Ig classes (including IgD on cord blood lymphocytes, cf. p. 39). Antisera specific for the terminal heavy chain domain (pFc′ cf. p. 34) stain more weakly suggesting attachment to the membrane through this region.

In some circumstances, a proportion of T-cells do stain for surface immunoglobulin. This is not a product of the T-cell itself but is acquired by adsorption and probably represents immune complexes binding to receptors for Ig Fc region which

FIGURE 3.6. (a) Stimulation of cortical lymphoid follicle with formation of germinal centre in draining lymph node six days after the induction of antibody synthesis by pneumococcus polysaccharide SSS III injected into the ear of a mouse. Plasma cells appear in the medulla. There is no cellular proliferation in the paracortical (thymus dependent) area.

(b) Stimulation of lymphoblasts in the paracortical area of the draining lymph node three days after the induction of a cell-mediated immuno-logical response to the contact sensitizer oxazolone applied to the ear. The primary nodules in the cortex are not stimulated.

(c) Lack of response in paracortical area in draining node of neonatally thymectomized mouse 3 days after application of oxazolone to the ear skin.

gc: germinal centre   pn: primary nodule
tda: thymus-dependent area
(Photographs kindly provided by Drs. M. de Sousa and D.M.V. Parrott.)

are displayed by *activated* T-cells. These can be demonstrated by the formation of rosettes with red cells coated with IgG antibody; clusters of red cells surround the lymphocyte to which they bind through the Fc of the coating IgG. In contrast, most if not all B-cells carry Fc receptors and form these 'Fc-rosettes' (figure 3.7a). In addition, approximately one half of the B-lymphocytes and a small proportion of T-cells form clusters with red cells coated with the third component of complement (C3; cf. 121) (Figure 3.7b).

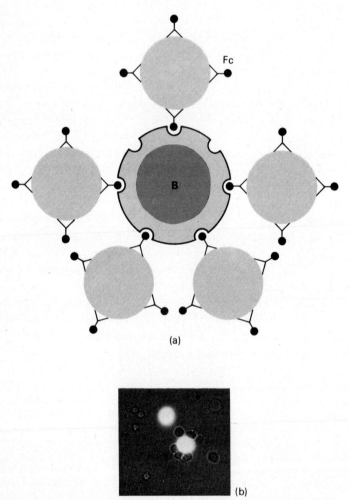

(a)

(b)

FIGURE 3.7. B-cell rosettes—(a) diagrammatic representation of rosette formed with IgG (Y) coated erythrocytes binding to the receptor for Fc (b) cluster of C3 coated red cells around B-lymphocyte (visualized in u.v. light after staining with acridine orange). (Courtesy of Dr. A. Arnaiz-Villena.)

Interestingly, human T-cells can be persuaded to form so-called 'spontaneous' rosettes with uncoated sheep erythrocytes, a useful if fortuitous reaction without any immunological foundation. The T-lymphocyte membrane also possesses a specific discriminating antigen which is shared by brain. In the mouse this is recognized as the θ iso-antigenic system (watch for the modern nomenclature—Thy. 1!) which is acquired as the cells differentiate within the thymus gland.

At the time of writing, the most popular means of enumerating lymphocyte populations in human blood is to use fluorescent anti-immunoglobulin for B-cells and spontaneous rosette formation for T-cells. Values given by these two tests usually add up to a few per cent short of 100%; without giving anything away, the remaining lymphocyte-like cells, negative on both counts, are termed 'null-cells'.

For the unwearying seeker after truth, the plot diversifies. Aside from the implication above that B-cells may exist as subpopulations, only one of which bears a C3 receptor, Raff has presented a case for two subpopulations of T cells in the mouse. T_1 which are essentially spleen seeking, relatively rich in θ and insensitive to anti-lymphocyte serum, and T_2 which migrate preferentially to lymph nodes, have little surface θ antigen and are comparatively sensitive *in vivo* to anti-lymphocyte serum. T_1 cells disappear quite rapidly after adult thymectomy (another piece of evidence showing that the thymus doesn't give up in adult life despite a considerable degree of involution). A subpopulation of human T-cells can now be distinguished by its reaction with a cold IgM autoantibody found by Thomas in the sera of certain patients with infectious mononucleosis, SLE and cold agglutinin disease. Clarification of the function of these cellular subsets is awaited.

B- and T-cells can be separated by electrophoresis, by selective depletion of one or the other by rosette formation and by affinity chromatography. In the latter, B-lymphocytes can be selectively retained on Sephadex columns to which anti-light chain is bound covalently, the effluent providing a T (+null-cell) population virtually free of Ig-bearing B-cells; the column-bound cells can be released by digestion of the support with dextranase (Schlossman and Hudson). In the latest model, the antibody is separated from the Sephadex by a 'spacer' molecule and bound cells can be recovered by comparatively gentle mechanical means.

LYMPHOCYTE SURFACE PHENOMENA

When viable B-lymphocytes are stained in the cold with a fluorescein-conjugated anti-Ig, the fluorescence is seen as patches on the cell surface (figure 3.8a). However, if the experiment is repeated using monovalent (Fab) anti-Ig, a smooth ring of surface fluorescence is observed (figure 3.8b). The interpretation of these findings is that the lymphocyte surface immunoglobulins are floating freely in the plasma membrane (like icebergs in a sea of lipid) and are agglutinated into little

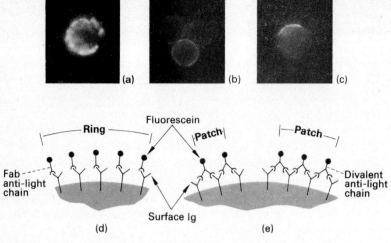

Figure 3.8. Patterns of immunofluorescent staining of B-lymphocyte surface immunoglobulin using fluorescein-conjugated anti-Ig (cf. p. 113 for discussion of technique). Provided the reaction is carried out in the cold to prevent pinocytosis, the labelled antibody cannot penetrate to the interior of the viable lymphocytes and reacts only with surface components. (a) patch formation with conjugated anti-Ig; (b) ring staining with monovalent (Fab) anti-Ig; (c) cap formation on warming the cells in (a); (d) diagram of ring staining by monovalent anti-Ig; (e) diagram of patch formation by divalent anti-Ig. (Photographs kindly provided by Drs. A. Arnaiz-Villena and L. Hudson.)

patches by the divalent anti-Ig (figure 3.8d and e). If the lymphocytes are now allowed to warm up, the patches coalesce to form a cap over one pole of the cell (figure 3.8c) and the complexes are taken into the cytoplasm by endocytosis leaving the surface free of immunoglobulin. The cell will resynthesize its surface immunoglobulin within a few hours if washed and incubated at 37° in fresh medium.

When rabbit lymphocytes are cultured in the presence of anti-Ig for a minimum of 16–20 hours, they go on to transform into blast-like cells (cf. figure 3.8) and divide. Activation also occurs with the divalent $F(ab')_2$ pepsin fragment derived from the anti-Ig but not the monovalent Fab with the strong implication that cross-linking and aggregation of surface Ig is an important step in B-lymphocyte stimulation. Current thinking however is that in most circumstances an additional 'nonspecific' signal is required for activation by antigen (Bretscher & Cohn).

Cellular co-operation in the immune response

THE ROLE OF MACROPHAGES

The large mononuclear cells of the monocyte-macrophage series play a central role in the induction of the immune response with respect to antigen presentation and may well prove to be capable of providing an accessory 'second signal'. Cytoplasmic contacts between macrophages and lymphocytes have been observed and co-operative effects of macrophages for antibody production are clearly revealed by tissue culture studies showing that the antibody response to most antigens is largely abrogated when glass-adherent cells are first removed from the responding lymphoid cell population, and that this defect can be overcome by the addition of macrophages. Furthermore, antigens such as bovine serum albumin provoke a vastly superior antibody response when injected together with macrophages rather than as a free solution; interestingly the more thymus-dependent the response to a given antigen, the greater the enhancing effect due to macrophages. Antigen trapping and concentration of antigen at the cell surface for effective presentation to the lymphocyte is a likely possibility. It is known for example, that antibody in a primed animal which is fixed to the surface of dendritic macrophages cupping cortical lymphoid follicles binds antigen efficiently (Nossal), and here presumably it is in a favourable location to stimulate a secondary response. Antigen taken up by free macrophages is partially degraded and partially fixed at or near the cell surface where it is thought to be in a strongly immunogenic state. The finding by Askonas and Rhodes that RNA prepared from these macrophages still contains antigen fragments and is highly immunogenic ('super-antigen') suggests that concentration alone is not the only mechanism by which stimulation is achieved and that a macrophage product (? RNA) unrelated to the specificity of the antigen is providing an accessory signal for lymphocyte activation. Account may also have to be taken of a possible role for Ig and C3 associated with antigen in immune complexes in view of Fc and C3 receptors on both cell types.

CO-OPERATION BETWEEN T- AND B-CELLS

We have already drawn attention to the fact that the antibody response to certain antigens is considerably depressed following neonatal thymectomy. However, we know from the work of Davies with chromosome (T6) marked thymus cells, that the T-lymphocytes do not themselves secrete antibody. This involvement of the T-lymphocyte in antibody synthesis without itself producing antibody is now seen to be due to a form of *co-operation* by the T-cell which helps the antigenic stimulation of B-lymphocytes to be more effective (figure 3.4). Using an irradiated mouse (which cannot itself make an immune response) as a 'living test-tube', Claman and his colleagues showed that thymocytes or bone marrow cells (containing B-cells) injected together with sheep red cells gave only poor or modest antibody production. When T- and B-cells were injected together, there was a very marked increase in the number of cells engaged in antibody synthesis (table 3.3).

The cellular origin of the antibody-forming cells was elegantly demonstrated by Miller and his colleagues in co-operation experiments involving transfer of T-cells and bone marrow from genetically different mouse strains. The antibody-forming cells in the recipient spleen were studied *in vitro* by the Jerne plaque technique (see below) and could be inhibited only by an antiserum to the transplantation antigens of the strain providing the bone marrow *not* the thymus cells (figure 3.9).

At the molecular level, further light on the nature of co-operation has been shed by the experiments of both Mitchison and Rajewsky who have shown that primed B-cells make a secondary antibody response to a hapten bound to protein carrier only when T-cells primed to the carrier ('helper cells') are also present (figure 3.10). In other words, when T-cells recognize and respond to carrier determinants, they help B-lymphocytes specific for the hapten to develop into antibody-forming cells (figure 3.11a). Mechanisms postulated to explain co-operation include (i) presentation of the hapten in a multivalent form to cross-link B-cell receptors (particularly when dealing with a molecule bearing a single hapten substituent

TABLE 3.3.

Irradiated recipient given antigen plus:	Antibody response
Spleen cells	+ + +
Thymocytes (T-cells)	±
Bone marrow (B-cells)	+
Thymocytes and bone marrow	+ + +

Co-operation of bone marrow and thymus cells in production of antibody to sheep red cells in irradiated recipient. (Note B-cells ≡ bursa equivalent and that T-cells are also derived from bone marrow before 'processing' by the thymus.)

60

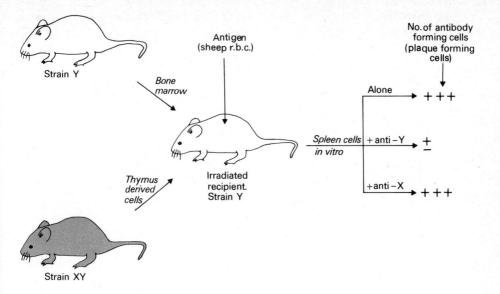

FIGURE 3.9. Bone marrow origin of antibody-forming cells. Antibody-forming cells were studied in the antigen stimulated recipient of a bone marrow/thymus mixture. Antibodies to the transplantation antigens of the strain providing bone marrow inhibited the plaque-forming cells whereas antibodies to the thymocyte donor were ineffective (based on Miller J.F.A.P. & Mitchell G.F., *J.exp.Med.* 1968, **128**, 821 : in these studies thymus derived cells from the thoracic duct were used).

which is effectively monovalent) (ii) a second signal independent of antigen which could be mediated through a T-lymphokine such as mitogenic factor (p. 151) or by a complex through the Fc and C3 receptors and (iii) some degree of amplification either by T-cell proliferation or by recruitment of macrophages by attachment of cytophilic antigen-specific receptors secreted by the T-lymphocytes. Some possible models are presented in figure 3.11 and it may be that several mechanisms will prove to be involved in the immune response *in vivo*, the contribution of each varying with the circumstances.

RELEVANCE TO ANTIGENICITY

When discussing the question of antigenicity in chapter 1 (p. 17) we were largely preoccupied with the factors governing the shape of the antigenic determinant and its fit with the antibody site without considering the initiation of an antibody response. If a single determinant binds to a B-lymphocyte surface receptor, no cross-linking will result (figure 3.12a) and the cell will not be activated (remember the definition of a hapten—

combines with antibody but won't stimulate antibody synthesis). Certain antigens which are highly polymeric with respect to a given determinant—pneumococcus polysaccharide, endotoxin, D-amino acid polymers and polyvinylpyrrolidine for example—are thymus independent and can stimulate B-cells directly. They bind with great avidity to the surface of the B-cell through their multivalent attachment (cf. p. 15) thereby cross-linking the surface receptors and stimulating the production of IgM but not IgG antibody; whether efficient cross-linking alone will trigger IgM-producing cells or whether these antigens provide a 'second signal' through the C3 receptor (by activating the alternate complement pathway; p. 122) or through some innate mitogenic capability is still open. Molecules which bear a smaller number of a given determinant cannot cross-link

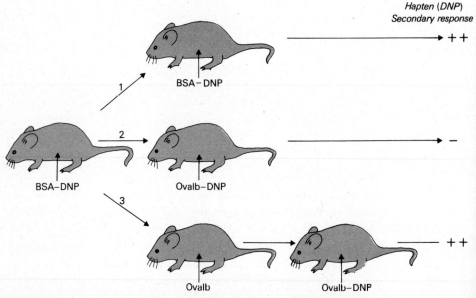

FIGURE 3.10. Carrier-hapten co-operation showing that a secondary response to the hapten (dinitrophenyl group—DNP) is only obtained when cells are primed to both carrier and hapten.

   1. After priming with an injection of DNP linked to bovine serum albumin (BSA) as a carrier, later inoculation with the same BSA–DNP combination gives a secondary response to DNP.

   2. If the primed animals are challenged instead with DNP on a different carrier, ovalbumin, there is no secondary response.

   3. However, if animals primed with BSA–DNP are further primed with ovalbumin, challenge with Ovalb–DNP will now give a secondary response. Similar results can be obtained using lymphoid cell transfers from primed animals into irradiated recipients. The 'helper-cells' with specificity for the carrier can be shown to be T-cells by the use of anti-θ serum or thymectomized donors.

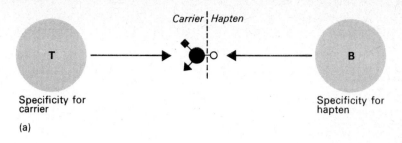

(a)

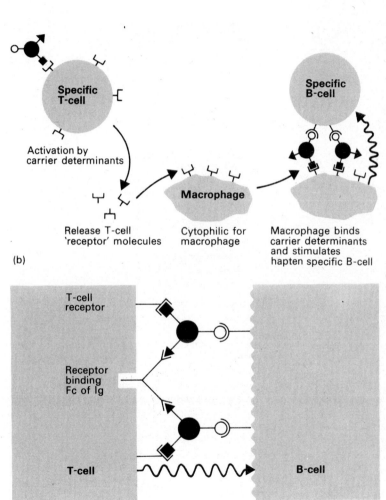

(b)

(c)

FIGURE 3.11. Some possible models for T-B co-operation.

(a) Carrier /hapten specificities

(b) Model I—macrophage presentation (Feldmann). C3 fixation by the complex on the macrophage may enhance the stimulus (Pepys)

(c) Model II—Antigen concentration and presentation by T-cells where it is held by specific T-cell receptors plus specific antibody binding to the

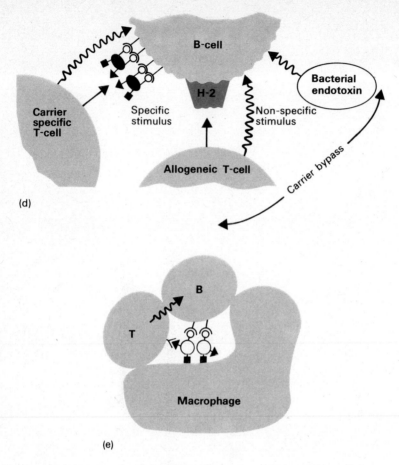

(d)

(e)

surface Fc receptor (the supposition being that the T-cell receptors are of too low a density and/or affinity to bind antigen effectively by themselves). (Playfair after Mitchison and Taylor.)

(d) Model III—Antigen binds to B-cell and the second signal is provided by a specific T-cell recognizing the carrier (Kreth and Williamson), by an allogeneic T-cell reacting with the surface histocompatibility determinants or by any other appropriate non-specific stimulus. Endotoxin only promotes IgM synthesis and cannot fully substitute for T-cells.

(e) Model IV—T and B cells interact with antigen which has bound to a macrophage non-specifically or specifically (through cytophilic antibody) (favoured by work of Askonas, Roelants, Unanue and Katz).

so efficiently and other determinants have to act as carriers by evoking T-cell co-operation. Such help from the T-cell must be even more essential for those cases where a determinant appears only once on each molecule (figure 3.12b) thereby acting in effect as a monovalent hapten. This will usually be the case with proteins which have little or no symmetry such as bovine serum albumin where it will be appreciated that each determinant can

64

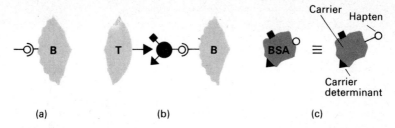

FIGURE 3.12. Response to a simple protein antigen looked at from the carrier-hapten standpoint. A small protein such as bovine serum albumin has several determinants but all are different, so that the molecule itself cannot cross-link B-cell receptors and behaves as a monovalent hapten with respect to each determinant (cf. (a)). Only if other determinants can be recognized by T-cells can appropriate co-operation be provided for B-cell stimulation (b). Thus the determinants on the protein act in a 'carrier' function for each other (c).

only activate its specific B-cell by calling upon the carrier function of the others (figure 3.12c). To a first approximation larger molecules tend to be better antigens because they have more determinants capable of acting as carriers. Where an animal lacks T-cells capable of recognizing potential carrier determinants, as for example in certain 'poor responder' strains (p. 85), there will be a correspondingly poor response to the hapten even if hapten-specific B-cells are present.

The overall picture is still admittedly uncertain. Very tentatively it might be said that cross-linking by multivalent antigens can trigger cells to produce IgM but that antigens which cross-link less effectively require a second signal. Where the second signal is provided by a T-cell (and this normally requires carrier determinants), a switch to IgG antibody synthesis can occur but in all other cases so far studied, help from the accessory signal is restricted to IgM production.

Synthesis of humoral antibody

DETECTION OF ANTIBODY-FORMING AND ANTIGEN-SENSITIVE CELLS

Immunofluorescence

Cells containing antibody within their cytoplasm can be identified by the 'sandwich' technique (see chapter 5). For example, a cell making antibodies to tetanus toxoid if treated with the antigen will then fix a fluorescein labelled anti-tetanus antibody and can be visualized as a specifically fluorescing cell in the ultraviolet microscope.

Plaque techniques

In the original technique developed by Jerne and Nordin, the cells from an animal immunized with sheep erythrocytes are suspended together with an excess of sheep red cells in agar. On incubation the antibody-forming cells release their immunoglobulin which coats the surrounding erythrocytes. Addition of complement (chapter 5) will then cause lysis of the coated cells and a plaque clear of red cells will be seen around each antibody-forming cell (figure 3.13). Direct plaques obtained in this way largely reveal IgM producers since this antibody had a high haemolytic efficiency. To demonstrate IgG synthesizing cells it is necessary to increase the complement binding of the erythrocyte-IgG antibody complex by first adding a rabbit anti-IgG serum; this develops the 'indirect plaques' and can be used to enumerate cells making antibodies in different immunoglobulin subclasses, provided the appropriate rabbit antisera are available. The method can be extended by coating an antigen such as pneumococcus polysaccharide onto the red cell, or by coupling hapten groups to the erythrocyte surface.

Rosette techniques

When lymphocytes are incubated with, say, sheep red cells, those with surface receptors for the erythrocytes will bind them to form a rosette (figure 3.14a). On more prolonged incubation, lymphoid cells which are secreting antibody become surrounded by a 'cluster' of erythrocytes (figure 3.14b). This technique, termed immunocytoadherence by Biozzi, can be modified by using red cells from different species or by coating different antigens onto isologous erythrocytes. Another variation involves the adherence of bacteria to the appropriate antigen-sensitive lymphocytes.

Both B- and T-lymphocytes can form rosettes and are inhibited from so doing by prior addition of an anti-light chain serum. On incubation in culture for several hours, B-cells retain the ability for rosette formation but T-cells lose theirs suggesting that the Ig-like receptor for erythrocytes was only loosely bound as might be expected if it were acquired as a cytophilic antibody (cf. 55). In support of this view is Cooper's observation that T-cells in a bursectomized chicken will only form

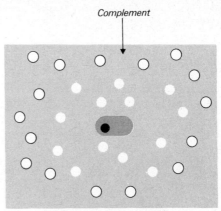

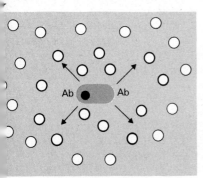

Secreted antibody coats
surrounding red cells

Coated erythrocytes lysed
on adding complement to
form plaque with antibody –
forming cell at centre.

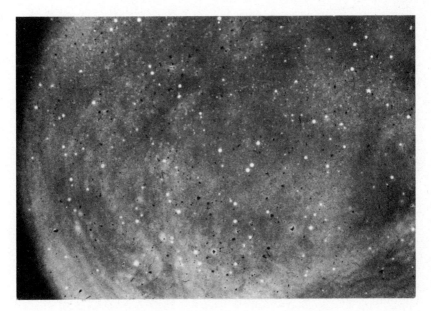

FIGURE 3.13. Jerne plaque technique for antibody-forming cells.

(a) The direct technique for cells synthesizing IgM haemolysin is shown.
The indirect technique for visualizing cells producing IgG haemolysins
requires the addition of anti-IgG plus complement in the final stage. The
difference between the plaques obtained by direct and indirect methods
gives the number of 'IgG' plaques.

(b) Photograph of plaques in agar plate (courtesy of Dr. J.H.L.
Playfair). Plaques show as small circular light areas.

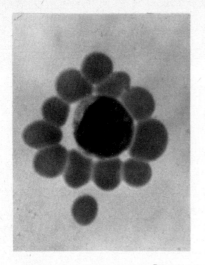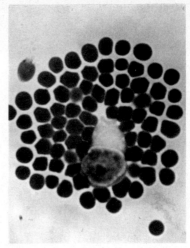

FIGURE 3.14. Immunocytoadherence technique.

(a) Mouse spleen cell forming a rosette with sheep red blood cells which are bound by the specific surface receptors. Cytocentrifuged preparation.

(b) Cluster formation by antibody-forming cells in the same preparation. The secreted antibody binds further erythrocytes to the central rosette (courtesy of F. Hay and L. Hudson).

rosettes with sheep erythrocytes if anti-sheep cell antibody is injected.

Focus formation

After transfer of relatively small numbers of lymphoid cells to an irradiated recipient, antigen challenge will produce foci of antibody forming cells which appear to be derived from single antigen-sensitive lymphocytes.

PROTEIN SYNTHESIS

In the normal antibody-forming cell there is a rapid turnover of light chains which are present in slight excess. Defective control occurs in many myeloma cells and one may see excessive production of light chains or complete suppression of heavy chain synthesis. Interchain disulphide bridges may form while the heavy chains are still attached to the ribosomes (figure 3.15) but the sequence in which the intermediates arise varies with the nature of the immunoglobulin. Using 'pulse and chase' techniques with radioactive amino acids it was found that the build-up of both light and heavy chains proceeds continuously starting from the N-terminal end. Furthermore, isolation of the

68

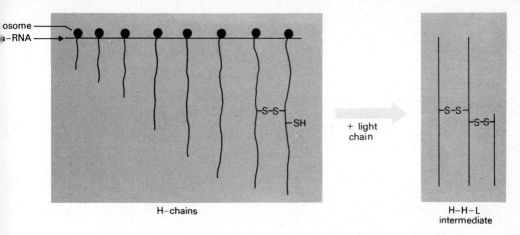

osome ——
ι–RNA ——→

—S—S—

—SH

+ light
chain

—S—S—

—S—S—

H–chains

H–H–L
intermediate

FIGURE 3.15. Synthesis of mouse IgG2a immunoglobulin. As the H-chains near completion, adjacent peptide chains can spontaneously cross-link through their constant regions. It is thought that the light chains may aid release of the terminal chains from the ribosome by forming the L—H—H molecule. Combination with a further light chain would yield the full immunoglobulin L—H—H—L (based on Askonas B.A. & Williamson A.R., *Biochem.J.* 1968, **109**, 637). The order in which the interchain disulphide bridges are formed varies in different immuno-globulins depending on the relative strengths of the bonds as assessed by susceptibility to reduction.

mRNA for each type of chain has shown them to be of appropriate size to allow synthesis of the complete peptides. The evidence is therefore against the view that either chain can be formed by joining together two preformed lengths of peptide and it is likely that the DNA sequence encoding the variable and constant regions of each chain is transcribed as one cistron. Stevens and Williamson have made the fascinating observation that heavy chain mRNA can bind specifically to immuno-globulin molecules from a variety of different species but the role of this interaction in control of transcription and translation is not yet clear.

IMMUNOGLOBULIN CLASSES

The synthesis of antibodies belonging to the various immuno-globulin classes proceeds at different rates. Usually there is an early IgM response which tends to fall off rapidly. IgG antibody synthesis builds up to its maximum over a longer time period. On secondary challenge with antigen, the time course of the IgM response resembles that seen in the primary though the peak may be higher. By contrast the synthesis of IgG antibodies rapidly accelerates to a much higher titre and there is a relatively slow fall-off in serum antibody levels (figure 3.16). The same probably holds for IgA and in a sense both these immuno-globulin classes provide the main *immediate* defence against future penetration by foreign antigens.

Antibody synthesis in certain classes shows considerable dependence upon T-co-operation in that the responses in T-deprived animals are strikingly deficient; such is true of mouse IgG1, IgE and part of the IgM antibody responses and of IgM memory. Complete Freund's adjuvant (p. 153) seems to act partly through stimulation of T-cells and thereby stimulates

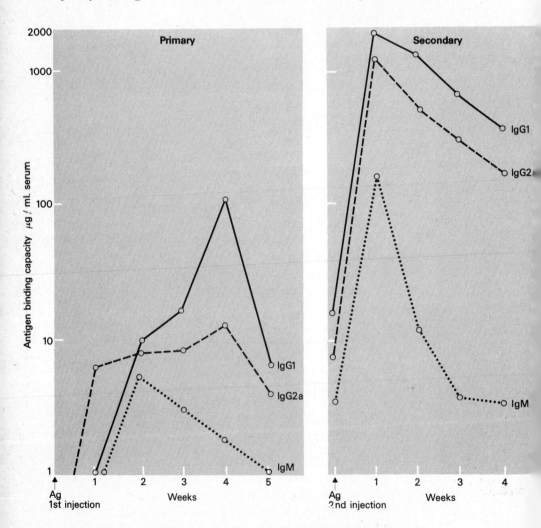

FIGURE 3.16. Synthesis of antibodies in different mouse immunoglobulin classes during the primary and secondary responses to bovine serum albumin. With agglutination techniques which greatly favour the detection of IgM, synthesis of this antibody class is apparent much earlier. (Data kindly provided by Dr. G. Torrigiani.)

antibody production in T-dependent classes. The prediction from this that the response to T-independent antigens (e.g. pneumococcus polysaccharide p. 62) should not be potentiated by Freund's adjuvant is borne out in practice; furthermore, as would be expected, these antigens evoke primarily IgM antibodies and poorly defined immunological memory as do T-dependent antigens injected into thymectomized hosts. Thus in rodents at least the switch from IgM to IgG appears to be under some degree of thymus or T-cell control. Another class-specific effect which must be mentioned is the tremendous enhancement of IgE responses by helminths and even by soluble extracts derived from them.

REGULATION OF THE ANTIBODY RESPONSE

Feedback mechanisms must operate to limit antibody production otherwise after antigenic stimulation we would become overwhelmed by the responding clones of antibody forming cells and their products, a clearly unwelcome state of affairs as may be clearly seen in multiple myeloma where control over lymphocyte proliferation is lost. Both Moller and Uhr have demonstrated that injection of preformed IgG antibody can inhibit the response to antigen suggesting that such antibodies synthesized *in vivo* must exert a homeostatic effect on the overall response. The simplest interpretation is that the antibody blocks antigenic determinants needed to drive continued lymphocyte stimulation. Alas this is only part of the story because $F(ab')_2$ antibodies are far less effective than whole IgG in switching off the reaction. In some way T-cells may be implicated; not only can they potentiate responses through co-operation but under other circumstances they can exert a suppressive function. For example: (a) adult thymectomy increases the response to 'T-independent' antigens and prevents the switch-off of IgE antibody to haptens coupled with Ascaris extracts (b) thymocytes from a young New Zealand Black (NZB) mouse can suppress autoantibody formation when injected into older diseased animals and (c) T-cells can sometimes transfer tolerance (see p. 165–6).

The prevention of Rh sensitization by administration of anti-D to mothers at risk (p. 139) is a good example of regulatory control by antibody. This feedback mechanism may also complicate the immunization of infants in those cases where appreciable levels of maternally derived IgG antibodies are present.

Antigenic competition, the name given to the phenomenon in

71

which injection of one antigen may inhibit the concurrent immune response to another immunologically unrelated antigen operates through the T-lymphocyte since only thymus-dependent antigens can be involved. The mechanism is unclear but competition can be of major importance in vaccination programmes where more than one antigen is being administered.

ABNORMAL IMMUNOGLOBULIN SYNTHESIS

In chapter 2 we discussed the production of unique monoclonal immunoglobulins in multiple myeloma where there is an uncontrolled proliferation of a single clone of Ig-producing plasma cells. IgG, IgA, IgD and IgE myeloma has been reported in frequencies which parallel their serum concentration; Waldenström's macroglobulinaemia represents a closely comparable situation involving monoclonal IgM production. The myeloma or 'M' component in serum is recognized as a tight band on paper electrophoresis (all molecules in the clone are of course identical and have the same mobility) and as an abnormal arc on immunoelectrophoresis with a 'bump' caused by the monoclonal protein (figure 3.17a and b). 'M' bands have been found in the sera of a number of individuals who have no clinical signs of myeloma; the comparative rarity with which

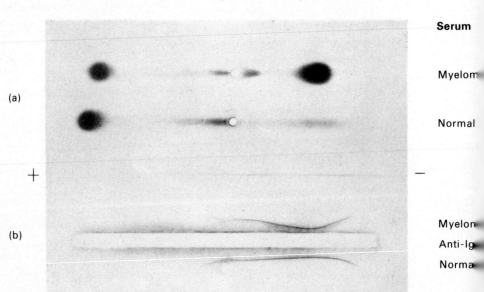

FIGURE 3.17. Myeloma serum with an 'M' component. (a) Agar gel electrophoresis showing strong band in γ-globulin region. (b) Immuno-electrophoresis against anti-IgG serum revealing the 'bump' or 'bow' in the precipitin arc. (Courtesy Dr. F.C. Hay.)

invasive multiple myeloma develops in these people and the constant level of the monoclonal protein over a period of years suggests the presence of benign tumours of the lymphocyte-plasma cell series.

Heavy chain disease is a rare condition in which quantities of abnormal heavy chains are excreted in the urine- γ-chains in association with malignant lymphoma and α-chains in cases of abdominal lymphoma with diffuse lymphoplasmacytic infiltration of the small intestine. The amino acid sequences of the N-terminal regions of these heavy chains are normal but they have a deletion extending from part of the variable domain through most of the C_{H1} region so that they lack the structure required to form cross-links to the light chains. One idea is that the defect arises through faulty coupling of V and C region genes (cf. p. 98).

ONTOGENY OF THE IMMUNE RESPONSE

The first signs of lymphopoiesis in utero appear by about three months in the human and are seen in the foetal liver and the thymus. The foetal liver (and later the bone marrow) is the source of stem cells which provide the lymphocytic component of the thymus. Lymph node and spleen remain relatively under-developed even at birth except where there has been intra-uterine exposure to antigens as in congenital infections with rubella or other organisms. The ability to reject grafts and to mount an antibody response is reasonably well developed by birth but the immunoglobulin levels with one exception are low particularly in the absence of intra-uterine infection. The exception is IgG which is acquired by placental transfer from the mother. This material is catabolized with a half life of approximately 30 days and there is a fall in IgG concentration over the first three months accentuated by the increase in blood volume of the growing infant. Thereafter the rate of synthesis overtakes the rate of breakdown of maternal IgG and the overall concentration increases steadily. The other immunoglobulins do not cross the placenta and the low but significant levels of IgM in cord blood are synthesized by the baby (figure 3.18). IgM reaches adult levels by nine months of age. Trace levels of IgA, IgD and IgE are present in the circulation of the newborn.

In the embryonic chick bursa, some of the lymphocytes switch their surface Ig from IgM to IgG and double labelling techniques reveal some cells with both together. Injection of anti-μ (anti-IgM heavy chain) into the embryo prevents the development of IgM and IgG producing cells whereas anti-γ inhibits only IgG development.

73

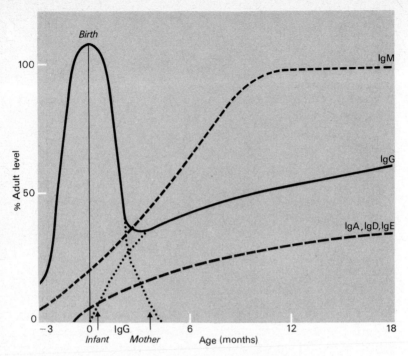

FIGURE 3.18. Development of serum immunoglobulin levels in the human (after Hobbs J.R. in *Immunology & Development*, ed. M. Adinolfi, 1969, p. 118. Heinemann, London).

PHYLOGENY OF THE IMMUNE RESPONSE

It has long been known that natural defence mechanisms such as phagocytosis occur in invertebrates. More recently it has become clear that bactericidins may be induced in the haemolymph of species like the lobster by infection with different gram negative and positive bacteria. The bactericidins can reach a maximum in one to two days with peak titres of 1 : 100 or more. They show broad reactivity in that they can kill bacteria antigenically unrelated to the inducing organism; characterization of these molecules to see if they are related in any way to vertebrate immunoglobulins is awaited with interest. With respect to cell-mediated immune reactions, there are now reports that the earthworm can develop transplantation immunity to tissues of the same or other species while permanently accepting autografts (i.e. grafts of its own tissue). An understanding of the nature of these cellular and humoral responses will surely provide some insight into whether the cellular reaction is really the most primitive in evolutionary terms.

All vertebrates are capable of generating an immunological

74

response on antigenic stimulation. Both B- and T-cell responses can be elicited even in the lowliest vertebrate studied, the California hagfish. This unpleasant cyclostome (which preys upon moribund fish by entering their mouths and eating the flesh from the inside) was originally considered 'the negative hero of the phylogeny of immunity' since unlike the lamprey, a more advanced cyclostome, it appeared incapable of reacting immunologically. It now transpires that hagfish can make antibodies to haemocyanin and reject allografts, provided they are maintained at temperatures approaching $20°$ (in general poikilotherms make antibodies better at higher temperatures). The antibodies were present in a $28S$ macroglobulin fraction, but further up the evolutionary scale in the cartilaginous fishes well-defined $18S$ and $7S$ immunoglobulins with heavy and light chains have now been defined.

It is worthy of note that the thymus is lymphoid in the bony and cartilaginous fishes but in the lamprey there is no clear indication of a lymphoid thymus although a primitive epithelial organ has been recognized. So far there has been no definite evidence of thymus tissue in the hagfish although a small round cell with a thin rim of basophilic cytoplasm found in peripheral blood may be a candidate for an 'early lymphocyte'.

One could imagine the way in which immunoglobulins might have evolved from enzymes. Take for example an enzyme which has as its substrate a sugar common to the surface of many types of bacterium. The enzyme will bind to the substrate molecule on the bacterial surface using the same forces which are involved in antigen-antibody interactions. If mutation in the enzyme molecule were to produce a configuration capable of binding to a structure on the surface of a phagocyte (or if mutation changed the phagocyte so that it could bind the enzyme), we would have a bacterium-binding protein cytophilic for phagocytes which would thereby act as an opsonin to increase the rate of bacterial phagocytosis (cf. p. 162). Further mutations would lead to variations in the substrate (antigen)-recognizing portion and in the phagocyte-binding region giving molecules with different recognition specificities and a variety of biological functions.

Immunological tolerance

AT BIRTH

Over 20 years ago Owen made the intriguing observation that non-identical (dizygotic) twin cattle, which shared the same placental circulation and whose circulations were thereby linked, grew up with appreciable numbers of red cells from the other twin in their blood; if they had not shared the same circulation at birth, red cells from the twin injected in adult life would be rapidly eliminated by an immunological response. From this finding Burnet conceived the notion that potential antigens which reach the lymphoid cells during their developing immunologically immature phase in the perinatal period can in some way specifically suppress any future response to that antigen when the animal reaches immunological maturity. This, he considered, would provide a means whereby unresponsiveness to the body's own constituents ('self') could be established and thereby enable the lymphoid cells to make the important distinction between 'self' and 'non-self'. On this basis, any foreign cells introduced into the body around the perinatal period should trick the animal into treating them as 'self' components in later life and the studies of Medawar and his colleagues have shown that *immunological tolerance* or unresponsiveness can be artificially induced in this way. Thus neonatal injection of CBA mouse cells into newborn A strain animals suppresses their ability to immunologically reject a CBA graft in adult life (figures 3.19 and 3.20). Tolerance can also be induced with soluble antigens; for example, rabbits injected with bovine serum albumin at birth fail to make antibodies on later challenge with this protein.

IN THE ADULT

It is now recognized that tolerance can be induced in the adult as well as the neonate. Mitchison repeatedly injected mature mice with various doses of bovine serum albumin (BSA) and then examined their ability to give an antibody response on challenge with BSA in a highly antigenic form (in complete Freund's adjuvant—see p. 153). Surprisingly, mice given repeated low doses of BSA became tolerant and made no response to the final BSA challenge; mice on medium doses of BSA became sensitized and gave a good antibody titre on challenge while those on high BSA doses were unresponsive, i.e. tolerant (figure 3.21). Thus there is a 'low zone' and a 'high zone' for tolerance in terms of antigen predosage. Many substances are antigenic even at relatively low doses and the antibody so formed combines with antigen to prevent it inducing low-zone tolerance. However, if an immunosuppressive drug such as cyclophosphamide is given at the same time to inhibit antibody synthesis, tolerance to these antigens is more readily established in the adult.

Elegant studies by Weigle and coworkers have pinpointed the

76

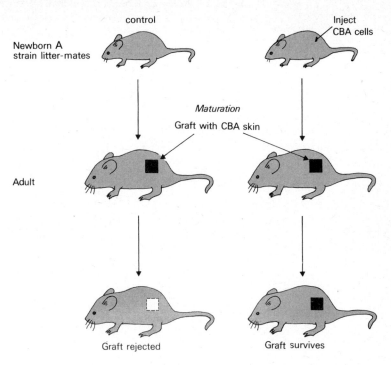

FIGURE 3.19. Induction of tolerance to foreign CBA skin graft in A strain mice by neonatal injection of antigen (after Billingham R., Brent L. & Medawar P.B.).

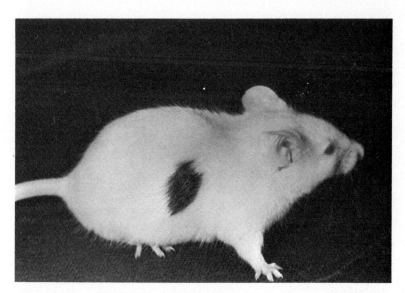

FIGURE 3.20. CBA skin graft on fully tolerant A strain mouse showing healthy hair growth eight weeks after grafting (courtesy of Professor L. Brent).

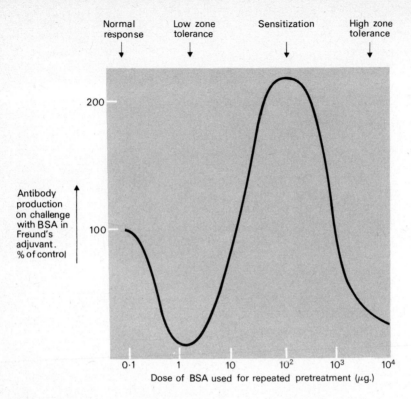

FIGURE 3.21. Production of low- and high-zone tolerance in mice by repeated injection of different doses of bovine serum albumin (BSA). Tolerance was then tested by inoculating the animals with BSA in a highly antigenic form in adjuvant (after Mitchison N.A., *Immunology* 1968, **15**, 509).

T-cell as the target for tolerance at low antigen levels while both B- and T-lymphocytes are made unresponsive at high antigen dose. For 'thymus-dependent' antigens at dose levels where the T-cells play a major co-operative role in antibody formation, the overall immunological performance of the animal will reflect the degree of reactivity of the T-cell population (table 3.4). The greater difficulty in making B-cells tolerant might be related to the higher concentration of surface receptors, but the kinetics of tolerance induction (figure 3.22) indicate not only that B-cells more rapidly regain responsiveness, but also that the mechanism of induction may be different. Thus there is evidence that T-cells from tolerant animals may play an active role in suppressing B-lymphocytes as shown by their ability to inhibit antibody formation after transfer to normal recipients (Gershon's 'infectious tolerance'). The facilitation of tolerance induction by cyclophosphamide, mentioned above, could be

TABLE 3.4. Effect of antigen dose on tolerance induction in
T- and B-cells

mg tolerogen administered	% Tolerance induced		
	T-cells	B-cells	Donor spleen
0·1	96	9	62
0·5	99	56	97
2·5	99	70	99

After induction of tolerance to aggregate-free human IgG in mice, the reactivity of
thymocytes and bone marrow cells (containing B-cells) was assessed by transfer to
irradiated recipients with either bone marrow or thymus respectively from normal
donors. The degree of tolerance induced in the donor is shown in the final column. Low
antigen doses tolerize the T-cells. B-cells become unresponsive at higher doses. The
T-cell activity largely dictates the response of the spleen as a whole (from Chiller J.M.,
Habicht G.S. & Weigle W.O., *Science*, 1971, **171**, 813).

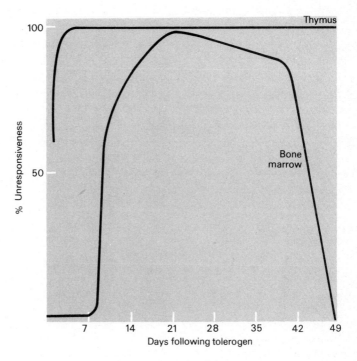

FIGURE 3.22. Kinetics of the induction of unresponsiveness in thymus and
bone-marrow (assumed to be B-) cells following tolerogenic dose of human
IgG in the mouse. T-cells are rapidly made tolerant and remain so.
B-cells more slowly reach their unresponsive state but the cell population
soon regains reactivity. (J. Chiller, G. Habicht and W.O. Weigle, *Science*,
1971, **171**, 813.) Subsequent studies have shown that *splenic* B-cells
become unresponsive more rapidly (< 3 days) but otherwise parallel the
bone marrow cells in their behaviour.

79

due to its cytotoxic effect on antigenically stimulated dividing B-cells, which would otherwise be difficult to render unresponsive.

Antigens are more tolerogenic (able to induce tolerance) when in a soluble rather than an aggregated or particulate form which can be readily taken up by macrophages. This has led to the suggestion that molecules are tolerogenic if they react directly with lymphocytes but antigenic if they are first processed by macrophages before presentation to the lymphocyte.

TERMINATION OF TOLERANCE

It will be remembered that a CBA skin graft will survive on an A strain animal made tolerant with CBA cells given at birth. Injection of normal adult A strain lymphoid cells into these animals will cause rejection of the CBA graft; the injected cells recognize the CBA skin as foreign because they are taken from a mouse which had not been artificially conditioned at birth to accept CBA antigens as self. Following these findings, Gowans showed that small lymphocytes obtained from the thoracic duct of a normal animal would abrogate the tolerant state and cause graft rejection but significantly, small lymphocytes from *tolerant* donors were not effective, *i.e. the small lymphocyte population has the power to be tolerant to or react against foreign antigens.*

In Medawar's experiments the tolerant state persisted for a long time because the living CBA lymphoid cells injected at birth continually divided and persisted. This cannot happen with non-living antigens such as BSA and in fact tolerance to neonatally administered BSA is gradually lost. One explanation is that new immunocompetent cells are constantly being recruited throughout life and in the absence of antigen are not rendered tolerant. Since recruitment of newly competent T-lymphocytes is drastically curtailed by removal of the thymus, it is of interest to note that the tolerant state persists for much longer if the animals are thymectomized.

When tolerance to a hapten is induced by injection of a hapten carrier we are probably concerned essentially with unresponsiveness of the T-cells since they are more readily tolerizable than B-cells; in other words carrier stimulated T-cell co-operation for triggering of hapten-specific B-cells is lost. This may be overcome:

(a) by injecting the hapten on a new carrier for which the animal has responsive T-cells. Such a mechanism may well account for the ability of cross-reacting antigens to break tolerance and could be of importance in relation to the production of autoantibodies by certain bacteria which share antigenic determinants with the host (cf. p. 223).

(b) by directly providing the second signal to the B-cell by stimulation with bacterial endotoxins or allogeneic T-cells (cf. the carrier bypass in figure 3.11d).

80

Further reading

Adinolfi M. (ed.) (1969) *Immunology and Development*. Spastics Int. Med. Publications, London.

Bevan M.J., Parkhouse R.M.R., Williamson A.R. & Askonas B.A. (1972) Biosynthesis of immunoglobulins. *Progress in Biophysics & Mol.Biol.*, **25**, 131.

Burnet F.M. (1969) *Self and Non-self*. Cambridge University Press.

Feldmann M. (1972) Cell interactions in the immune response *in vitro*: V, Specific collaboration via complexes of antigen and thymus-derived cell immunoglobulin. *J.exp.Med.*, **136**, 737.

Feldmann M. & Nossal G.J.V. (1972) Cellular basis of antibody production. *Quart.Rev.Biol.*, **47**, 269.

Greaves M.F., Owen J. & Raff M. (1973) T & B lymphocytes: their origins, properties and roles in immune responses. North Holland, Amsterdam.

Hildemann W.H. & Reddy A.L. (1973) Phylogeny of immune responsiveness: marine invertebrates *Fed.Proc.*, **32**, 2188.

Kreth H.W. & Williamson A.R. (1971) Cell surveillance model for lymphocyte co-operation. *Nature*, **234**, 454.

Nossal G.J.V. (1973) The cellular and molecular basis of immunological tolerance. *Essays in Fundamental Immunology 1*, page 28. Blackwells Scientific Publications, Oxford.

Playfair J.H.L. (1971) Cell co-operation in the immune response. *Clin.exp. Immunol.*, **8**, 839.

Porter, Ruth & Knight, Julie (1972) *Ontogeny of Acquired Immunity*. Ciba Foundation Symposium. Elsevier, Amsterdam.

Stevens R.H. & Williamson A.R. (1973) Translational control of H-chain synthesis. *J.Mol.Biol.*, **78**, 505 and 517.

Watson J., Trenkner E. & Cohn M. (1973) The use of bacterial lipopolysaccharides to show that two signals are required for the induction of antibody synthesis. *J.exp.Med.*, **138**, 699. (Note that these authors do not consider cross-linking of receptors to be a necessary condition for induction.)

Weigle W.O. (1973) Immunological Unresponsiveness. *Adv. in Immunology*, **16**, 61.

4 Theories of antibody synthesis

Instructive theory

The ability of animals to synthesize antibodies directed against determinants such as dinitrobenzene and sulphanilic acid, which were so unlikely to occur in nature, made it difficult to accept the idea based on Ehrlich's earlier views that the body has preformed antibodies whose production is further stimulated by the entry of antigen. Instead attention turned to theories in which the antigen acted instructively as a template around which a standard unfolded γ-globulin chain could be moulded to provide the appropriate complementary shape. The molecule would be stabilized in this configuration by disulphide linkages, hydrogen bonds and so forth; on separation from the template the molecule would now have a specific combining site for antigen (figure 4.1).

Selective theory

An alternative view holds that the information required for the synthesis of the different antibodies is already present in the genetic apparatus. The gene which codes for a specific antibody is selected and 'switched on' by contact of antigen with the cell, and through transcription and translation of the appropriate messenger RNA, immunoglobulin peptide chains with corresponding individual primary amino acid sequences are synthesized; based on the sequence, these chains then fold spontaneously to a preferred globular configuration which possesses the specific antigen-combining sites (figure 4.1).

An analogy may help in the comparison of these two theories. If we consider the purchase of a suit, two courses of action are open. We may *instruct* the tailor to make the suit to measure, in which case we act as a template for the suit to be made on. Alternatively the tailor may be an enterprising fellow who has already made up 10^4 different suits, one of which is almost certain to fit any intending purchaser; all we have to do is *select* the best fit for ourselves. Although in both cases the know-how

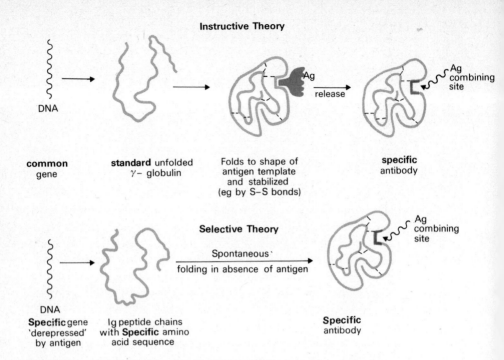

Instructive Theory

DNA

common
gene

standard unfolded
γ- globulin

Folds to shape of
antigen template
and stabilized
(eg by S-S bonds)

Ag

release

Ag
combining
site

specific
antibody

Selective Theory

Spontaneous
folding in absence of antigen

Ag
combining
site

DNA
Specific gene
'derepressed'
by antigen

Ig peptide chains
with Specific amino
acid sequence

Specific
antibody

FIGURE 4.1. Comparison of instructive and selective theories for generating specific antigen-combining site.

of making suits (cf. protein synthesis) is there, in the first instance we provide essential information for the final shape (as the antigen does), whereas in the second situation the tailor himself had the ability to make a whole variety of differently shaped suits (information already in the DNA) before seeing the customer (antigen).

Evidence for a selective theory

ABSENCE OF ANTIGEN FROM PLASMA CELLS

Using autoradiography to visualize highly radioactive antigens combined with immunofluorescence to identify cells making specific antibody, Nossall has shown that nearly all cells which contain intracellular antibody do not have demonstrable antigen molecules. This is clearly at variance with the idea of antigen acting as a template.

84

UNFOLDING EXPERIMENTS

Reduction of disulphide bonds in IgG or its Fab fragment followed by treatment with high concentrations of guanidine effectively destroys any organized secondary structure. However, removal of the guanidine from the unfolded molecules by dialysis and reoxidation restores significant specific antigen-binding activity. This is inconsistent with the instructive view (which requires the presence of antigen for the formation of a specific antibody) and indicates that the information held in the primary amino acid sequences is sufficient to allow the correct tertiary structure to be formed by spontaneous refolding. An analogous result has been obtained with ribonuclease; after unfolding, the molecule can spontaneously recover its enzymic activity.

AMINO ACID SEQUENCE OF ANTIBODIES

Purified antibodies show differences in amino acid sequence. As mentioned previously, myeloma proteins which represent individual immunoglobulin molecules show considerable variability in the sequences of the N-terminal part of both light and heavy chains. Indeed of the many human myeloma light chains so far sequenced, none have proved to have identical structures. These differences in amino acid sequence reflect differences in DNA nucleotide sequences strongly implicating genetic control of specificity.

GENETIC STUDIES

Immune responsiveness to certain defined antigens has indeed been linked to genetic constitution, in particular with genes controlling the synthesis of major transplantation or histocompatibility antigens (see chapter 8). Thus mice of the $H-2^b$ group all respond well to the synthetic polypeptide antigen TGAL (a polylysine backbone with side chains of polyalanine randomly tipped with mixed tyrosine and glutamyl residues), whereas mice of $H-2^a$ specificity respond poorly. With another synthetic antigen (HGAL, having histidine in place of tyrosine) the position can be reversed, the 'poor TGAL responders' now giving a good antibody response and the 'good TGAL responders' a weak one showing that the capacity of a given strain to give a high or low response is not a general characteristic but varies with the individual antigen in question. This ability to respond

85

well or poorly segregates as though it were a single gene chromosomally linked to but not identical with H-2. In fact, studies on recombinant H-2 alleles derived from known genetic crossovers locate the so-called *immune response (Ir) gene* within the H-2 pseudolocus and specifically between those regions encoding the Ss and the H-2K antigens (cf. p. 185). The Ir gene appears to be expressed through the activity of the T-cells. For example although high and low responders to TGAL have comparable numbers of antigen-specific B cells, the poor responders give only low affinity IgM antibody and a poor secondary response whereas good responders give high affinity IgG antibody and well-developed memory unless T-deprived when they behave as do the poor responders. The ability to mount an antibody response to low doses of different T-dependent antigens also shows H-2 linkage, while in guinea pigs, genetically-linked immune responsiveness to poly-L-lysine (PLL) is associated with the ability of PLL to act as a good carrier for haptens.

An agreeable hypothesis is that the Ir gene product is itself the specific T-cell receptor (cf. 149) and that a series of Ir genes provide a variety of T-cell specificities by coding for a defined spectrum of different 'variable regions' (? each linked to a 'constant region' expressing the major transplantation antigen).

The immune response can be influenced by genetic factors in other quite different ways as instanced by the low responder Biozzi mice which have a genetically linked macrophage defect.

Clonal selection model

The evidence clearly favours a genetic theory and we should now examine how this can be expressed in cellular terms. Clonal selection, based largely on the ideas elaborated by Burnet, is generally regarded as an acceptable working model for antibody synthesis.

It is envisaged that each lymphocyte has the genetic information available to make one particular antibody and molecules of that antibody are built into the cell-surface membrane as receptors. Different lymphocytes have different antibodies so that all the body lymphocytes between them present antibodies with a wide spectrum of specificities. Antigen will combine with those lymphocytes carrying antibody on their surface which is a good fit, and these cells will be stimulated by the reaction on the plasma membrane to differentiate and divide to form a clone of cells synthesizing antibody with the same specificity as that on the surface of the parent lymphocyte (figure 4.2).

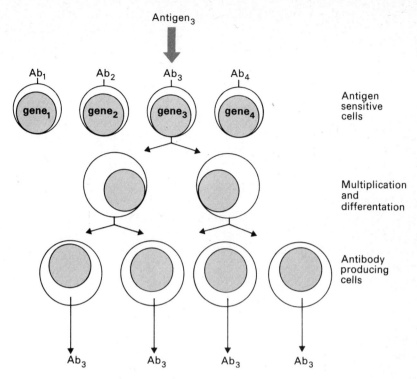

FIGURE 4.2. Clonal selection model. Each lymphocyte has the genes coding for one specific antibody, several molecules of which are built into the surface membrane to act as receptors. In the diagram, antigen$_3$ combines with the cell capable of making the complementary antibody$_3$ and this reaction at the cell surface leads to the formation of a clone of daughter cells making and exporting that specific antibody.

Some of the progeny revert to small lymphocytes and become memory cells.

Evidence for clonal selection model

ONE CELL/ONE IMMUNOGLOBULIN

With immunofluorescent techniques, immunoglobulin-producing cells can be stained for either κ- or λ-chains but not both, and in the heterozygous rabbit, for the maternal allotypic marker or the paternal but never both together (*allelic exclusion*). Furthermore plasma cell tumours only produce one, and not more than one, myeloma protein. Similar restrictions apply to the staining of surface Ig on B-lymphocytes described in the last chapter (p. 58).

87

That these surface immunoglobulins can behave as antibodies is suggested by the ability of a small percentage of lymphocytes to bind specific antigens such as sheep cells (forming 'rosettes') or radioactive salmonella flagellin. This binding can be blocked by anti-immunoglobulin sera. Humphrey has further shown that the percentage of cells binding antigen is increased in primed and decreased in tolerant animals.

When a soluble antigen like polymerized flagellin binds to a specific cell it causes patching and capping of the surface Ig in just the same way as an anti-Ig serum (cf. p. 58). If the antigen-capped cells are now stained with fluorescent anti-Ig, all the Ig is found in the cap, there being none on the remainder of the lymphocyte surface, i.e. when antigen reacts with a cell, all the Ig molecules on the cell surface combine with the antigen showing that they have similar specificity. In summary, the surface Ig of each B-lymphocyte represents the product of only one of the two chromosomes which code for Ig and behaves as antibody of a single specificity.

RELATION OF SURFACE ANTIBODY TO
FUTURE PERFORMANCE

When cells are taken from an animal which has given a primary response to both ovalbumin and bovine serum albumin (BSA) and are passed down a column of glass beads coated with BSA, they retain the ability to give a secondary antibody response to ovalbumin but are unresponsive to BSA. Thus the BSA-responsive cells have anti-BSA receptors on their surface which cause them to stick to the BSA-coated beads (figure 4.3).

Other investigations have shown that cells primed for a humoral secondary response can be inhibited if treated with anti-immunoglobulin serum before the second contact with antigen. One may conclude that the surface antibody plays a key role in the recognition of antigen for the triggering of the lymphocyte response.

The evidence concerning the one cell/one antibody model cited above probably relates to committed primed B-lymphocytes but whether 'virgin' uncommitted lymphocytes express more than one specificity is still an unresolved question. Furthermore, there are isolated pieces of evidence, e.g. some studies of cells from animals immunized with more than one determinant and results of certain graft vs. host experiments, which would be consistent with multiple specificities (of T-cells in the latter case), but their interpretation is still uncertain. At this stage it is simpler to postulate one antibody for each cell so that *specific* combination with antigen at the surface generates a *non-specific* signal to the interior which initiates differentiation and proliferation. If there were two or more antibodies on the cell surface it is more difficult to construct a mechanism by which the cell would know which antibody had reacted. Difficult but not impossible. Suppose a virgin cell expresses two surface Ig specificities—one coded for by the paternal, the other by the maternal chromosome. Specific antigen reacts with one of them and the cell divides still making both Ig's. At some stage during this antigen induced differentiation, the cell must switch to one or other of the specificities because we know that B-lymphocytes ultimately show allelic exclusion. If exclusion is random, half the cells opting for production of relevant antibody will still be driven to proliferate by antigen and they will then predominate over the other cells which soon cease division through lack of antigen stimulation.

Validity of the clonal selection model

Antibody affinity and antigen dosage

The combination of antigen and antibody is reversible and the complex may readily dissociate, depending upon the strength

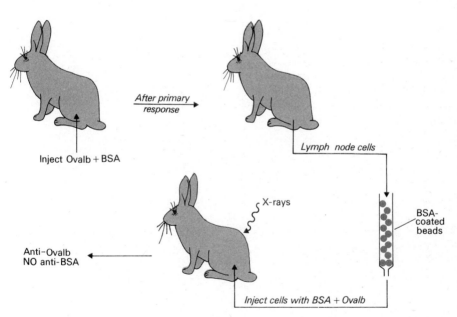

After primary response

Lymph node cells

Inject Ovalb + BSA

X-rays

BSA-coated beads

Anti-Ovalb
NO anti-BSA

Inject cells with BSA + Ovalb

FIGURE 4.3. Absorption of antibody-forming cell precursors on antigen coated column. Lymph node cells primed to ovalbumin (ovalb) and bovine serum albumin (BSA) are run down a column of BSA-coated glass beads and injected into an irradiated recipient. On secondary challenge anti-ovalb but no anti-BSA is produced showing that the cells destined to make anti-BSA were bound to the column presumably through their specific anti-BSA receptors on the surface. (Based upon the work of Wigzell H. & Anderson B., *J.exp.Med.* 1969, **129**, 23.)

of binding. This can be defined broadly through the equilibrium constant of the reaction:

$$Ag + Ab \rightleftharpoons AgAb$$

and the reactants will behave according to the laws of mass action (cf. chapter 1, p. 12). If the antigen and antibody fit together very closely, the equilibrium will lie well over to the right; we refer to such antibodies which bind strongly to the antigen as *high-affinity antibodies* (strictly *high avidity* in the case of multivalent antigens, cf. p. 15). Experimentally it is found that injection of *small* amounts of antigen leads to the production of *high*-affinity antibodies whereas *larger* amounts of antigen gives more antibody of *lower* affinity. How can we account for this on the clonal selection model?

It may be supposed that when an appropriate number of antigen molecules are bound to the antibody receptors on the cell surface, the lymphocyte will be stimulated to develop into an antibody-producing clone. When only small amounts of antigen are present, only those lymphocytes with high-affinity antibody receptors will be able to bind sufficient antigen for stimulation to occur and their daughter cells will, of course, also produce high-affinity antibody. Consideration of the antigen–antibody equilibrium equation will show that as the concentration of antigen is increased, even antibodies with relatively low affinity will bind more antigen; therefore at high doses of antigen the lymphocytes with lower affinity antibody receptors will also be stimulated and, as may be seen from figure 4.4, these are more abundant than those with receptors of high affinity.

Feedback inhibition of antibody synthesis

It was mentioned above (p. 71) that the injection of preformed antibody could inhibit an immune response to antigen and that this suggests a possible negative feedback model for control of antibody synthesis *in vivo*. The higher the affinity of the injected IgG antibody used to inhibit the immune response, the more effective it is. On the basis of the clonal selection model it may be argued that there will be a competition between injected antibody and the lymphocyte receptors for antigen and only cells with receptors of higher affinity than the administered antibody will be triggered. The higher the affinity of the antibody, the smaller will be the percentage of the total cells available (cf. figure 4.4).

90

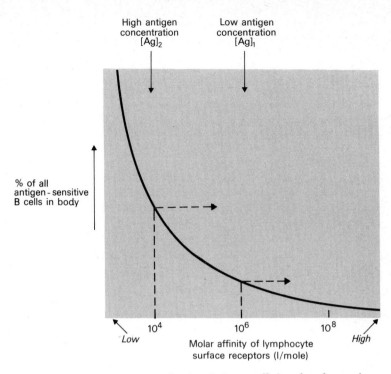

FIGURE 4.4. Antigen concentration in relation to affinity of surface anti-body receptors on lymphocytes which are stimulated. A certain antigen concentration $[Ag]_1$ will lead to binding of sufficient antigen molecules to lymphocytes bearing receptors of affinity 10^6 litre/mole and higher to cause stimulation; assuming the cells will synthesize the same antibody as that present on their surface, the antibodies so produced will thus have affinity of 10^6 litre/mole and higher. At a much higher antigen concentration $[Ag]_2$, lower affinity receptors will now be capable of binding the requisite number of antigen molecules to be triggered. Thus the antibodies produced will now be of affinity 10^4 litre/mole and higher, but as the cell distribution curve shows that the number of cells capable of synthesizing the low-affinity antibodies is much greater, the resulting antiserum will consist predominantly of these low-affinity immunoglobulins.

Increase of affinity during immunization

As immunization proceeds, only lymphocytes with higher and higher affinity receptors can be triggered because the concentration of available antigen steadily falls and feedback inhibition by synthesized antibody will 'turn off' cells with equal or lower affinity receptors.

Relative affinities of IgM and IgG

If we take IgM and IgG antibodies with antigen-binding sites of identical magnitude, the IgM molecules would have a far greater ability to bind antigen (avidity) than IgG; the ratio of the avidities would be disproportionately greater than the ratio of the combining valencies due to the 'bonus' effect of multivalency on avidity (cf. p. 15). On this basis we would expect IgM surface receptors of *low affinity* to bind as many antigen molecules as IgG receptors of *higher affinity* (i.e. the low-affinity IgM would have the same avidity as high-affinity IgG). If these receptors are on different cells then in response to a given dose of antigen, the IgM produced would be of lower affinity than the IgG. The experimental observations of Makaela are consistent with these predictions of the clonal selection model.

Hapten inhibition of antibody synthesis

Mitchison has found that if lymphoid cells are taken from a mouse primed with a hapten-carrier complex, treated *in vitro* with excess of free hapten and then transferred to an irradiated recipient, they fail to give a secondary response to the hapten carrier injected simultaneously. This inhibition by free hapten is ascribed to its binding to lymphocyte surface receptors so making them unavailable for reaction with the antigen hapten-carrier complex. When a cross-reacting hapten is used for the inhibition step, the final antiserum produced gives reasonably good binding with the homologous hapten but very poor cross-reaction, i.e. the hapten used for inhibition had selectively suppressed the reactivity of those cells with which it was best able to combine.

Effect of net charge of the antigen

Rabbit IgG antibodies can be separated by ion exchange chromatography into two major fractions, in one of which the proteins have a greater net positive charge than in the other. Antigens with a net negative charge favour the synthesis of the more positively charged antibodies and *vice versa* (Sela & Mozes). This would be fully consistent with the preferential binding of antigens to cells with surface receptors of opposite charge, other factors being equal.

Immunological tolerance

The clonal selection model readily provides a basis for the mechanism of tolerance induction. It has only to be postulated that under the conditions known to cause unresponsiveness, contact with antigen causes death or long-term inactivation of the antigen-sensitive cell rather than its stimulation. Although we are uncertain of the mechanism, the idea that deletion of specific clones is responsible for tolerance induction is attractive.

92

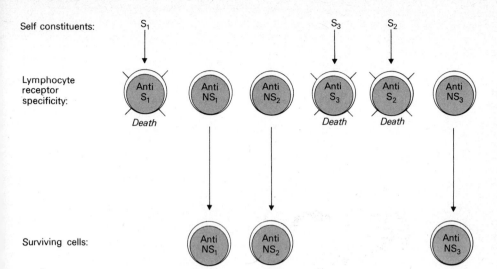

Self constituents:

Lymphocyte receptor specificity:

Surviving cells:

FIGURE 4.5. Induction of tolerance to self-constituents (S_1-S_3) by selective elimination of lymphocytes with self-reacting surface receptors. These cells are either killed or inactivated. Surviving cells are able to react only with non-self (NS) foreign antigens of specificity NS_1, NS_2, NS_3 etc.

For example, it can account for the development of self-tolerance since all lymphocytes having receptors capable of reacting with circulating or accessible self-components would be eliminated leaving only those cells with receptors for non-self determinants in the immunological armamentarium (figure 4.5).

Other experimental models of tolerance induction would appear to work on similar principles. Lymphoid cells treated *in vitro* with a very highly radioactive antigen selectively lose their ability to respond to the unlabelled form of the antigen on transfer to an irradiated host; this suggests that the antigen-sensitive lymphocytes bound labelled antigen to their surface and were killed or at least prevented from dividing by intense irradiation from the radioisotope. Another approach is through the selective deletion of B-cells carrying one allotype by injection of antiallotype serum in hetero-zygous animals. The antiallotype serum reacts with the surface receptors close to the antigen-combining site and behaves like antigen in causing lymphocyte stimulation under some circumstances, e.g. in tissue culture and suppression in others, e.g. injection at birth. It is remarkable that allotype suppression is maintained by T-cell control and that T-cells from such animals can suppress the expression of that allotype by B-cells from normal mice. It may well be profitable to ask whether this model provides a basis for understanding other situations which lead to suppression, such as the inhibitory effects of anti-μ in chick embryos (p. 73) and in particular the establishment of tolerance to self-antigens—all involving interaction of the inhibitory agent, be it antibody or antigen, with receptors of the cell destined for suppression.

93

One highly speculative possibility for inactivation or diversion of self-reacting clones would be a form of allelic switch. Let us suppose a lymphocyte expresses self-reactivity; combination with self antigen at a given phase in the cell's life history might trigger a switch to use an immunoglobulin-coding allele on the other chromosome. If this is of non-self specificity the cell would relax. If the new specificity was still self-reacting, the cell could switch back to the first chromosome but this time using a different V gene and so on.

Genetic theories of antibody variability

The variation in primary amino acid sequence of different antibodies, the differences between animal strains in their immunological responsiveness to selected synthetic and viral antigens and the plausibility of the clonal selection model all speak for a genetic basis underlying antibody variability. Similarities in amino acid sequence (homology) between the loops formed by intrachain disulphide bonds in the constant parts of heavy and light chains (figure 2.14) and to some extent between variable and constant parts, suggest that the existing genes controlling immunoglobulin structure are derived from a primitive smaller gene—perhaps coding for a peptide half the length of a light chain—by a process of duplication and translocation with early divergence of V genes.

Consideration of the percentage of lymphocytes capable of firmly binding defined labelled antigens and the proportion of normal mouse immunoglobulins reacting with an idiotypic antibody prepared against a myeloma protein, would lead one to guess very roughly that there may be something of the order of 10^4–10^5 different antibody specificities expressed in a single individual. What then is the genetic basis for this diversity of specificity? Approaches to this problem fall under two major headings (figure 4.6):

(a) *Somatic mutation.* It is envisaged that lymphocyte precursor cells carry a basic 'immunoglobulin' gene which, during differentiation, undergoes randomized somatic mutation with nucleotide changes in the DNA at certain susceptible positions. In this way the gene carried by one lymphocyte will differ from that in another so that the lymphocytes will each express different specificities.

(b) *Germ line.* The other view is that as a result of evolution all the genes coding for 10^4–10^5 different antibodies are present in the germ line and therefore are all contained in each lymphocyte.

Although it is difficult to decide between these two approaches, some comments may be made. The germ line theory,

94

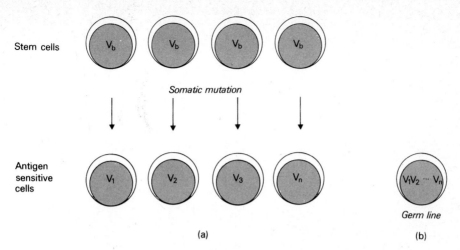

Stem cells

Somatic mutation

Antigen sensitive cells

Germ line

(a)

(b)

FIGURE 4.6. Somatic mutation and germ-line theories of antibody diversity: (a) a basic gene V_b undergoes somatic mutation during evolution from a stem cell to give different genes, one in each lymphocyte, coding for different antibodies with specificities from 1 to n; (b) each lymphocyte has the full range of genes coding for specificities 1 to n but only expresses one of these genes when stimulated by antigen.

if it employs 10^5 genes, would involve a large part of the DNA of one chromosome although some may think this a fair price to pay for the advantages of having an immunological system of wide specificity. However, with the evolution of both heavy and light chains, each contributing to antibody specificity, the total number of genes required is far fewer. Assuming that all combinations of different heavy and light chains are possible, p genes coding for heavy chains and q genes coding for light chains will give $p \times q$ antibody specificities with a total of only $(p+q)$ genes. For example, suppose there were 1,000 genes coding for light and another 1,000 for heavy chains: the total number of genes would be 2×10^3 but the number of potential antibody specificities would be 10^6.

A more serious objection, certainly against *repeated* genes coding for the constant part of the chains, is the presence of genetic markers (allotypes) in this region of the immunoglobulin molecule; with a large number of repeating genes containing a genetic marker, crossing over during meiosis would be bound to occur leading to mixing of alleles on the same chromosome (figure 4.7). This does *not* occur since the allotypic markers are inherited as single Mendelian traits. This had led to the suggestion that the germ line contains all the genes coding for the *variable* parts of the different immunoglobulin chains (V genes) but only one set for the *constant* parts (C genes). Since

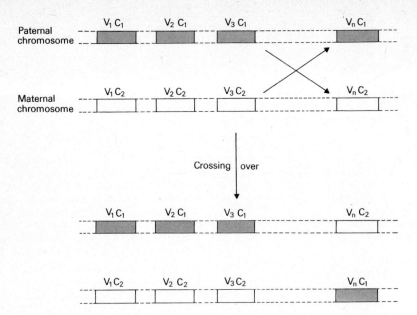

FIGURE 4.7. Showing how repeating the same allelic marker (either C_1 or C_2) in many genes along a chromosome would lead to ultimate mixing of the markers in the heterozygote by crossing over during meiosis. This does *not* happen with immunoglobulin allotypes since the markers segregate as single Mendelian factors, and it is therefore unlikely that the genes are repeated many times.

biosynthetic studies have shown that the immunoglobulin peptide chains are each synthesized as single units and not as two separate halves which are then joined together, it is most likely that the appropriate V and C genes must first combine to form a single ciston. The finding of myeloma proteins of different subclass but identical heavy chain V region amino acid sequence in the same patient and the presence of a similar idiotype (the antigenic determinant of the V region, cf. p. 41) on IgM and IgG antibodies in the same rabbit argues cogently for separate V and C region genes with the V gene switching from one C gene to another as the antibody class changes. Accepting the feasibility of combination between V and C genes, we still have a problem with the germ line theory if there is confirmation of reports that rabbit immunoglobulins show allotypic markers (the a locus) in the variable part of the heavy chain. The same considerations as before would make it unlikely that a V gene containing this a allele could be repeated many times and still segregate as a single Mendelian character unless some unusual mechanism is operating to prevent crossover. One may also be forced to postulate a special mechanism to conserve the full repertoire of V genes from erosion through genetic drift caused by random mutation in the germ line (although mutation at the hypervariable regions would be acceptable and even desirable).

Despite these objections there is a groundswell of opinion sympathetically inclined to a germ line view—and for some cogent reasons.

(1) The first relates to the existence of light chain subgroups. When the amino acid sequences of the variable part of human myeloma κ light chains are analysed, if one excludes the highly variable positions presumably linked to the antigen binding site, the remainder of the N-terminal region occurs in three quite different amino acid patterns (subgroups $V_{\kappa I}$, $V_{\kappa II}$, and $V_{\kappa III}$); each κ chain belongs to one of these three patterns, all of which are present in the serum of each individual (isotypic variation; p. 40). This would not be consistent with a single V gene undergoing random mutation and there must therefore be a minimum of three different V genes connected with the κ specificity. The same reasoning leads to the view that there are a minimum of a further five V genes associated with the λ specificity.

(2) But there is a further body of evidence which suggests that the number of genes in the germ line is much larger, and this is concerned with the finding of identical V region products expressed by different individuals. When animals are immunized so as to give an antibody response of restricted clonality (e.g. injecting DNP linked to Gramicidin S) many of the clones produced in different animals are identical on iso-electric focusing and many carry the same idiotypic determinant. Furthermore analysis of light chains from λ-myelomas produced in an inbred mouse strain showed 9/15 to be identical. Now 95% of mouse Ig are κ type and in contrast, only 2/50 κ Bence Jones light chains studied appeared to be the same. This would give a figure of the order of 700 V κ genes and a correspondingly lower number for λ genes. The variation in κ myelomas which occurs even in an inbred group, makes it likely that the failure so far to find identical myeloma proteins in different patients must be attributed to the outbred and heterozygotic nature of human populations.

In summary, a body of germ line V genes may provide the diversity of antibody response needed; somatic mutation could increase this variation further but there is as yet no evidence for its operation. Each lymphocyte becomes committed to the expression of one V_L and one V_H gene which combine with C region genes to provide an antibody of given specificity, class and type (figure 4.8). The cell posts immunoglobulin receptors

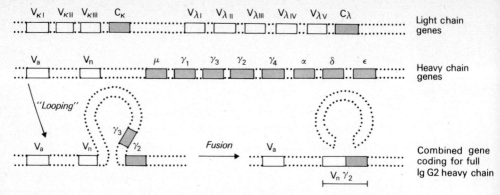

FIGURE 4.8. Hypothetical model for heavy and light chain genes. A number of V genes coding for variable sequences are present in the germ line including several for each of the light chain subgroups shown. There may then be translocation to a C gene coding for a constant region (in arbitrary order). Genes $V_{\kappa I-III}$ can link with the C_κ, $V_{\lambda I-V}$ with C_λ and V_a-V_n with one of the C genes coding for a heavy chain class or subclass. A possible 'looping' process in the DNA may be visualized. In the example shown the fused gene codes for V_n specificity linked in an IgG2 heavy chain.

with this specificity on its surface and if these are recognized by reaction with an antigen, clonal amplification and differentiation occurs to provide a large population of cells making antibody of the required specificity.

Further reading

Benacerraf B. & McDevitt H.O. (1972) Histocompatibility-linked immune response genes. *Science*, **175**, 273.

Fudenberg H.H., Pink J.R.L., Stites, D.P. & Wang A-C. (1972) *Basic Immunogenetics*. Oxford University Press, New York.

Hood L. & Prahl J. (1971) The immune system: a model for differentiation in higher organisms. *Adv. Immunol.*, **14**, 291.

Siskind G.W. & Benacerraf B. (1969) Cell selection by antigen in the immune response. *Adv. Immunol.*, **10**, 1.

Wigzell H. (1973) Antibody diversity: is it all coded for by the germ line genes? *Scand.J.Immunol.*, **2**, 199.

5

Interaction of antigen and antibody *in vitro*

Precipitation

QUANTITATIVE PRECIPITIN CURVES

Multivalent antigens mixed with bivalent antibodies in solution can combine to form three dimensional lattices which aggregate and precipitate. As described in chapter 1 (p. 4) the amount of precipitate varies with the proportions of the reagents and the following points were made:

(a) At 'equivalent' (optimal) proportions virtually all the antigen and antibody precipitate together and neither can be detected in the supernatant. From the weight of the precipitate, the antibody content of the serum can be calculated. Also at optimal proportions the most rapid precipitin formation is observed.

(b) In antibody excess, at least with most rabbit antisera, the complexes formed with antigen are insoluble; this allows an estimate of the antigen valency to be made.

(c) The precipitate tends to dissolve in antigen excess due to the formation of soluble complexes.

Certain horse and human antisera, particularly those directed against antigens with few determinants, differ in that they also form soluble complexes in *antibody* excess—partly because they are small and possibly also because of the relative solubility of horse and human immunoglobulins.

PRECIPITATION IN GELS

The precipitation reaction can be visualized in gels. In the double diffusion method of Ouchterlony, antigen and antibody placed in wells cut in agar gel, diffuse towards each other and precipitate to form an opaque line in the region where they meet in optimal proportions. A preparation containing several antigens will give rise to multiple lines (figure 5.1a). The immunological relationship between two antigens can be assessed by setting up the precipitation reactions in adjacent

99

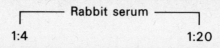

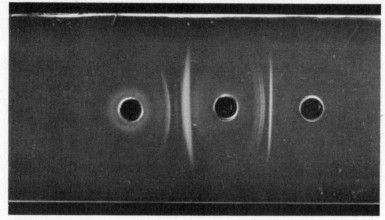

Goat anti-rabbit serum

(a)

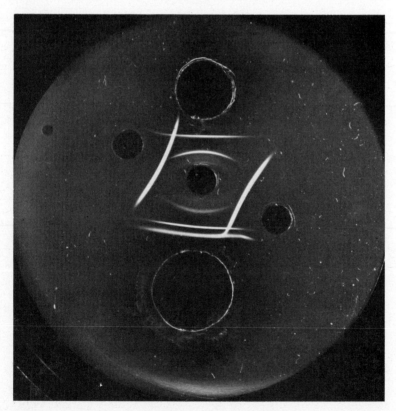

Antiserum in centre well

(b)

wells; the lines formed by each antigen may be completely confluent indicating immunological identity, they may show a
'spur' as in the case of partially related antigens, or they may
cross, indicative of unrelated antigens (figure 5.1b). The origins
of these patterns are explained in figure 5.2. It should be
emphasized that even in the case of confluent lines this can only
indicate immunological identity in terms of the antiserum used,
not necessarily molecular identity. For example, purified antibodies to the dinitrobenzene hapten would give a line of confluence when set up against dinitrobenzene–ovalbumin and
dinitrobenzene–serum albumin conjugates placed in adjacent
wells.

Where reagents are present in balanced proportions, the line
formed will generally be concave to the well containing the

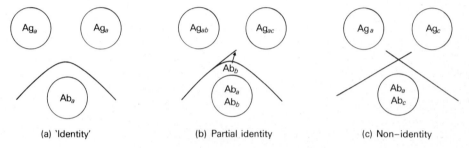

(a) 'Identity'   (b) Partial identity   (c) Non–identity

FIGURE 5.2. (a) Line of confluence obtained with two antigens which
cannot be distinguished by the antiserum used.

(b) Spur formation by partially related antigens having a common
determinant a but individual determinants b and c reacting with a mixture
of antibodies directed against a and b. The antigen with determinants a
and c can only precipitate antibodies directed to a. The remaining antibodies (Ab_b) cross the precipitin line to react with the antigen from the
adjacent well which has determinant b giving rise to a 'spur' over the
precipitin line.

(c) Crossing over of lines formed with unrelated antigens.

FIGURE 5.1a. Multiple lines formed in the Ouchterlony test (double-
diffusion precipitation) when rabbit serum and a goat anti-rabbit serum
react in agar gel. Since several distinct antigen–antibody systems are
present they clearly cannot all be present in balanced proportions. Where
they are, the line formed is sharp. Where there is gross imbalance the lines
become fuzzy and in the case of antigens which are present in considerable
excess, the precipitate obtained initially will redissolve due to the formation of soluble complexes and be pushed back towards the antiserum well.
This is clearly seen with the lines nearest the antibody well which are
indistinct at a rabbit serum dilution of 1:4, but are sharp when the antigen
is further diluted (courtesy of Dr. F.C. Hay).

FIGURE 5.1b. An Ouchterlony plate illustrating the antigenic relationships
between different preparations.

reactant of higher molecular weight, be it antigen or antibody. This is a consequence of the usually slower diffusion rate of larger sized molecules.

The gel precipitation method can be made more sensitive by incorporating the antiserum in the agar and allowing the antigen to diffuse into it; up to 90 per cent serum in agar may be employed (Feinberg). This method of single radial immuno-diffusion is used for the quantitative estimation of antigens.

SINGLE RADIAL IMMUNODIFFUSION
(SRID)

When antigen diffuses from a well into agar containing suitably diluted antiserum, initially it is present in a relatively high concentration and forms soluble complexes; as the antigen diffuses further the concentration continuously falls until the point is reached at which the reactants are nearer optimal proportions and a ring of precipitate is formed. The higher the concentration of antigen, the greater the diameter of this ring (figure 5.3). By incorporating, say, three standards of known antigen concentration in the plate, a calibration curve can be obtained and used to determine the amount of antigen in the unknown samples tested (figure 5.4). The method is used routinely in clinical immunology, particularly for immuno-globulin determinations, and also for components such as β_{1C}-globulin (third component of complement), transferrin, C-reactive protein and the embryonic protein, α-foetoprotein, which is associated with certain liver tumours.

IMMUNOELECTROPHORESIS

The principle of this has been described earlier (p. 28). The method is of value for the identification of antigens by their electrophoretic mobility, particularly when other antigens are also present. In clinical immunology, semi-quantitative infor-mation regarding immunoglobulin concentrations and identi-fication of myeloma proteins is provided by this technique.

There have been some felicitous developments of the prin-ciple combining electrophoresis with immunoprecipitation in which movement in an electric field drives the antigen directly into contact with antibody. *Crossover electrophoresis* may be applied to antigens which migrate towards the positive pole in agar (see figure 5.5). This qualitative technique is considerably more sensitive than double diffusion (Ouchterlony) and is used for the detection of hepatitis B antigen or antibody, and of anti-

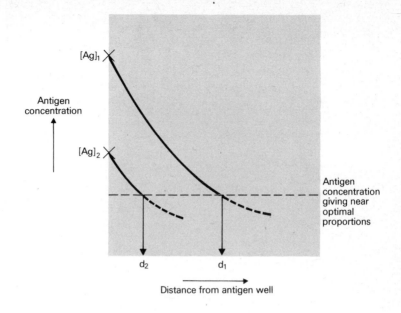

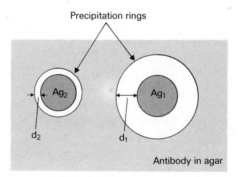

FIGURE 5.3. Single radial immunodiffusion: relation of antigen concentration to size of precipitation ring formed. Antigen at higher concentrations diffuses further from the well before it falls to the level giving precipitation with antibody near optimal proportions.

DNA antibodies in SLE (cf. p. 231). *Rocket electrophoresis* is a quantitative method which involves electrophoresis of antigen into a gel containing antibody. The precipitation arc has the appearance of a rocket, the length of which is related to antigen concentration (figure 5.6). Like crossover electrophoresis this is a rapid method but again the antigen must move to the positive pole on electrophoresis; it is therefore suitable for proteins such as albumin, transferrin and caeruloplasmin but immunoglobulins are more conveniently quantitated by single radial

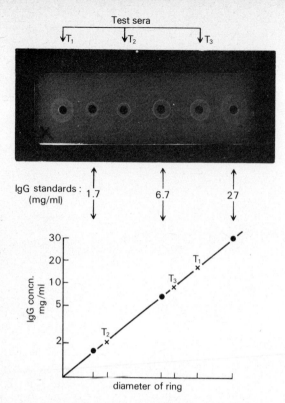

FIGURE 5.4. Measurement of IgG concentration in serum by single radial immuno-diffusion. The diameter of the standards (●) enables a calibration curve to be drawn and the concentration of IgG in the sera under test can be read off:

   T_1—serum from patient with IgG myeloma; 15 mg/ml

   T_2—serum from patient with hypogammaglobulinaemia; 2·6 mg/ml

   T_3—normal serum; 9·6 mg/ml.

(Courtesy of Dr. F.C. Hay.)

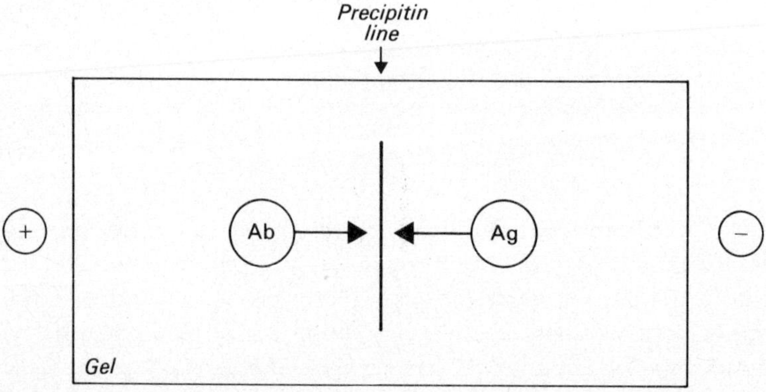

Precipitin line

```
(+)        Ab →   ←  Ag        (−)

     Gel
```

FIGURE 5.5. Cross-over electrophoresis. Antibody moves 'backwards' in the gel on electrophoresis due to endosmosis; an antigen which is negatively charged at the pH employed will move towards the positive pole and precipitate on contact with antibody.

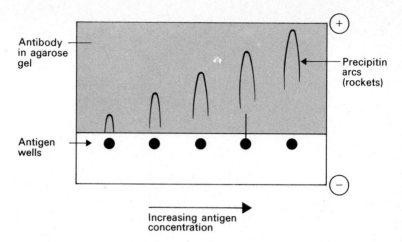

FIGURE 5.6. Rocket electrophoresis. Antigen is electrophoresed into gel containing antibody. The distance from the starting well to the front of the rocket shaped arc is related to antigen concentration.

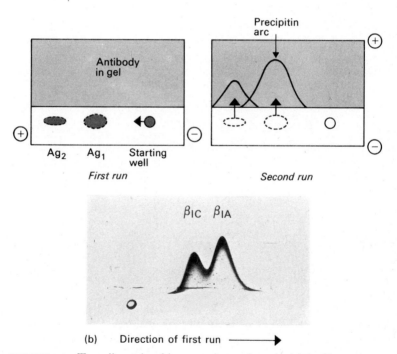

FIGURE 5.7. Two-dimensional immunoelectrophoresis. (a) Antigens are separated on the basis of electrophoretic mobility. The second run at right angles to the first drives the antigens into the antiserum-containing gel to form precipitin peaks; the area under the peak is related to the concentration of antigen. (b) Actual run showing C3 conversion ($\beta_{1C} \rightarrow \beta_{1A}$) in serum. In this case the arcs interact because of common antigenic determinants. (Courtesy of Dr. C. Loveday.)

105

immunodiffusion. One powerful variant of the rocket system, Laurell's *two-dimensional immunoelectrophoresis*, involves a preliminary electrophoretic separation of an antigen mixture in a direction perpendicular to that of the final 'rocket-stage' (figure 5.7a). In this way one can quantitate each of several antigens in a mixture. One straightforward example is the estimation of the degree of conversion of the third component of complement ($C3$;β_{1C}) to the inactive form β_{1A}(cf. p. 122 and 148) which may occur in the serum of patients with active SLE or the synovial fluid of affected joints in active rheumatoid arthritis, to give but two examples (figure 5.7b).

Antigen binding techniques

These methods assess antibody level either by determining the capacity of an antiserum to complex with radioactive antigen or by measuring the amount of immunoglobulin binding to an insoluble antigen preparation. Perhaps the point should be made that it is not possible to define the *absolute* concentration of antibody in a given serum because each serum contains immunoglobulins with a range of binding affinities and the estimation of the amount of antigen bound to antibody depends upon the concentration and affinities of the antibodies as well as the nature and sensitivity of the test. With this proviso, the quantitative tests described do give a measure of the antibody content of a serum which is of practical value.

DETERMINATION OF ANTIGEN-BINDING CAPACITY

The two methods to be considered involve the addition of excess radio-labelled antigen to the antiserum followed by assessment of the amount of antigen which has been complexed with antibody (this being the antigen binding capacity). This is achieved either by:

(a) *the Farr technique* in which complexed antigen is separated from that in the free form by precipitation with 50 per cent ammonium sulphate (only applicable to those antigens soluble at this salt concentration), or

(b) *the antiglobulin coprecipitation technique* in which the antigen bound to antibody is precipitated together with the rest of the immunoglobulin by an antiglobulin serum, leaving free antigen in the supernatant (figure 5.8). By using antibodies to different immunoglobulin classes and subclasses as the anti-

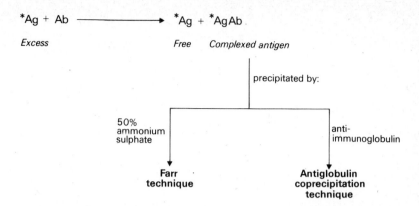

*Ag + Ab ⟶ *Ag + *AgAb

Excess   Free   Complexed antigen

precipitated by:

50%
ammonium
sulphate   anti-
                                           immunoglobulin

Farr   **Antiglobulin**
technique   **coprecipitation**
                                  technique

FIGURE 5.8. Determination of antigen-binding capacity. After addition of excess radioactive antigen (*Ag), that part bound to antibody as a complex is precipitated either by ammonium sulphate (Farr) or by an antiglobulin (antiglobulin coprecipitation).

globulin reagent, it is possible to determine the distribution of antibody activity among the classes. For example, addition of a radioactive antigen to human serum followed by a precipitating rabbit antihuman IgA, would indicate how much antigen had been bound to the serum IgA. The data documented in figure 3.16 on p. 70 were obtained by similar methods.

QUANTITATIVE IMMUNOADSORPTION

Antibody in a given volume of serum can be adsorbed onto antigen which has been made insoluble by cross-linking with reagents such as bisdiazobenzidine or glutaraldehyde. After washing to remove contaminants, the antibody can be released by lowering the pH and the antigen removed by centrifugation. All the protein present in the supernatant is now specific antibody and by estimating the content of different immunoglobulin classes by single radial immunodiffusion, the quantitative distribution of the antibody among the classes (and even subclasses) can be determined (figure 5.9). This method has proved useful for routine determination of antiglobulin factors in cases of rheumatoid arthritis.

A flexible variant is to estimate the antibody combined with the insoluble antigen by measuring the amount of radiolabelled anti-immunoglobulin that can be bound. The distribution of antibody in different classes can obviously be determined by using specific antisera. Take the radioallergosorbent test (RAST) for IgE antibodies in allergic patients. The allergen (e.g. pollen extract) is covalently coupled to a paper disc which

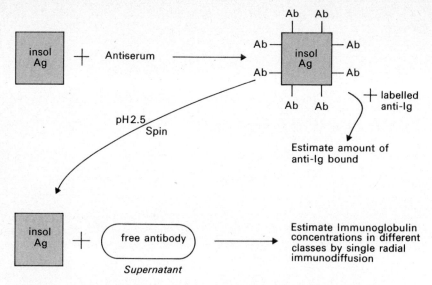

FIGURE 5.9. Principle of quantitative immunoadsorption technique for estimation of antibody. The antibody is isolated from the antiserum by adsorption onto insoluble antigen, released by acid and the amount of antibody immunoglobulin determined by single radial immunodiffusion using specific anti-immunoglobulin sera. Alternatively bound antibody may be determined by the ability to fix labelled anti-Ig. Class or sub-class specific antisera can be employed for this second stage.

is then treated with patient's serum. The amount of specific IgE bound to the paper is then estimated by addition of labelled anti-IgE.

RADIOIMMUNOASSAY

The binding of radioactively labelled antigen to a fixed amount of antibody can be partially inhibited by addition of unlabelled antigen and the extent of this inhibition can be used as a measure of the unlabelled material added. The principle is explained in figure 5.10. Methods vary in the means used to separate free antigen from that bound to antibody: some use coprecipitation of the complex with anti-immunoglobulin sera, others adsorption of free antigen onto charcoal and so on. With the development of methods for labelling antigens to a high specific activity, very low concentrations down to the 10^{-12} g/ml level can be detected and most of the protein hormones can now be assayed with this technique. One disadvantage is that these methods cannot distinguish active protein molecules from biologically inactive fragments which still retain antigenic determinants. Other applications include the radioimmuno-

	Free antigen	Bound antigen	Ratio free : bound radioactivity
(a) 150 *Ag + 100 Ab $\longrightarrow$	50 *Ag +	100 *Ag Ab	1:2
(b) 150 Ag + 150 *Ag + 100 Ab $\longrightarrow$	100 *Ag 100 Ag } +	{ 50 *Ag Ab 50 Ag Ab }	2:1

*Ag = radioactive antigen   Ag = unlabelled antigen

FIGURE 5.10. Principle of radioimmunoassay (simplified by assuming a very highly avid antibody and one combining site per antibody molecule).

(a) If we add 150 mol of radiolabelled Ag to 100 mol of Ab, 50 mol of Ag will be free and 100 bound to Ab. The ratio of the counts of free to bound will be 1 : 2.

(b) If we now add 150 mol of unlabelled Ag plus 150 mol radio Ag to the Ab, again only 100 mol of total Ag will be bound, but since the Ab cannot distinguish labelled from unlabelled Ag, half will be radioactive. The remaining antigen will be free and the ratio free : bound radioactivity changes to 2 : 1. This ratio will vary with the amount of unlabelled Ag added and this enables a calibration curve to be constructed.

sorbent test (RIST) for IgE, and the assay of carcinoembryonic antigen, hepatitis B (Australia) antigen and smaller molecules such as steroids and morphine-related drugs (appropriate antibodies are raised by coupling to an immunogenic carrier).

Immunofluorescence

Fluorescent dyes such as fluorescein and rhodamine can be coupled to antibodies without destroying their specificity. Coons showed that such conjugates would combine with antigen present in a tissue section and that the bound antibody could be visualized in the ultraviolet microscope through the emission of fluorescence. In this way the distribution of antigen throughout a tissue and within cells can be demonstrated. Looked at another way, the method can also be used for the detection of antibodies directed against antigens already known to be present in a given tissue section or cell preparation. There are three general ways in which the test is carried out.

1. Direct test

The antibody to the tissue substrate is itself conjugated with the fluorochrome and applied directly (figure 5.11a). For example,

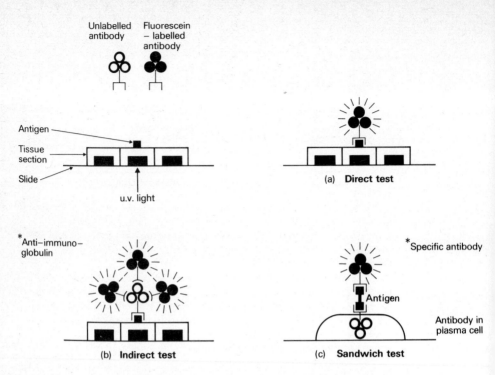

Unlabelled antibody   Fluorescein – labelled antibody

Antigen

Tissue section

Slide

u.v. light

(a) **Direct test**

*Anti–immuno–globulin

(b) **Indirect test**

*Specific antibody

Antigen

Antibody in plasma cell

(c) **Sandwich test**

FIGURE 5.11. Fluorescent antibody tests. *=fluorescein labelled.

suppose we wished to show the tissue distribution of a gastric autoantigen reacting with the autoantibodies present in the serum of a patient with pernicious anaemia. We would isolate IgG from the patient's serum, conjugate it with fluorescein, and apply it to a section of human gastric mucosa on a slide. When viewed in the u.v. microscope we would see that the cytoplasm of the parietal cells was brightly fluorescent.

2. *Indirect test*

The unlabelled antibody is applied directly to the tissue substrate and visualized by treatment with a fluorochrome-conjugated anti-immunoglobulin serum (figure 5.11b). To follow on from the above example, we can apply the indirect test to find out whether the serum of a patient has antibodies to gastric parietal cells. We would first treat a gastric section with patient's serum, wash well and then apply a fluorescein-labelled rabbit anti-human immunoglobulin serum; if antibodies were present, there would be staining of the parietal cells (figure 5.12a).

This technique has several advantages. In the first place the fluorescence is brighter than with the direct test since several

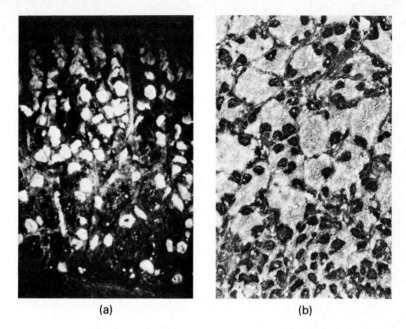

(a)   (b)

FIGURE 5.12. Staining of gastric parietal cells by (a) fluorescein and (b) peroxidase linked antibody. The sections were sequentially treated with human parietal cell autoantibodies and then with the conjugated rabbit anti-human IgG. The enzyme was visualized by the peroxidase reaction. (Courtesy of Miss V. Petts.)

fluorescent anti-immunoglobulins bind onto each of the antibody molecules present in the first layer (figure 5.11b). Secondly, since the conjugation process is lengthy, much time can be saved when many sera have to be screened for antibody because it is only necessary to prepare a single labelled reagent, viz. the anti-immunoglobulin. Furthermore, the method has great flexibility. For example, by using conjugates of antisera to individual immunoglobulin heavy chains, the distribution of antibodies among the various classes and subclasses can be assessed at least semi-quantitatively. One can also test for complement fixation on the tissue section by adding a mixture of the first antibody plus a source of complement, followed by a fluorescent anti-complement reagent as the second layer. Even greater sensitivity can be attained by using a third layer. Thus, in the example quoted of antibodies to parietal cells, we could treat the stomach section sequentially with the following: patient's serum containing antibodies to parietal cells, then a rabbit anti-human IgG, and finally a fluorescein-conjugated goat anti-rabbit IgG. However, as with most immunological techniques as *sensitivity* is increased, *specificity* becomes progressively reduced and careful controls are essential.

Applications of the indirect test may be seen in figure 5.12a and in chapter 9 (e.g. figure 9.2, pp. 215–6).

3. Sandwich test

This is a double layer procedure designed to visualize specific antibody. If, for example, we wished to see how many cells in a preparation of lymphoid tissue were synthesizing antibody to pneumococcus polysaccharide, we would first fix the cells with ethanol to prevent the antibody being washed away during the test, and then treat with a solution of the polysaccharide antigen. After washing, a fluorescein labelled antibody to the polysaccharide would then be added to locate those cells which had specifically bound the antigen (figure 5.11c). The name of the test derives from the fact that antigen is sandwiched between the antibody present in the cell substrate and that added as the second layer.

OTHER LABELLED ANTIBODY METHODS

In place of fluorescent markers, other workers have evolved methods in which enzymes such as peroxidase or phosphatase are coupled to antibodies and these can be visualized by conventional histochemical methods at both light microscope (figure 5.12b) and electron microscope (figure 5.13) level.

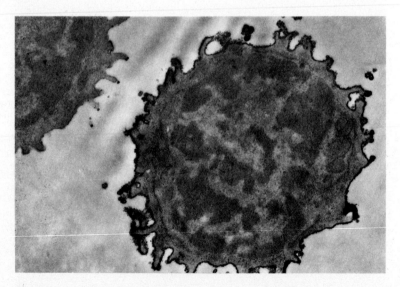

FIGURE 5.13. Electron microscopic visualization of human IgG on the surface of a B-lymphocyte by treatment of viable cell suspensions with peroxidase coupled anti-IgG. Note the adjacent unstained lymphocyte. (Courtesy of Miss V. Petts.)

Ferritin-conjugated antibody has also been used for ultra-structural localization of antigens; its distribution can be readily seen from its electron density and the characteristic tetrameric appearance of the iron core. An intriguing development designed originally for the demonstration of mouse iso-antigens in the electron microscope involves binding of mouse isoantibody to the cells followed by treatment with an artificially prepared hybrid antibody with dual specificity for mouse immunoglobulin and horse ferritin. Ferritin is then added as the final layer and is visualized in the electron microscope.

Reactions with cell surface antigens

BINDING OF ANTIBODY

Surface antigens can be detected and localized by the use of labelled antibodies. Because antibodies cannot readily penetrate within cells except by endocytosis, treatment of cells with labelled antibody in the cold (to minimize endocytosis) should lead to staining only of antigens on the surface. Such studies have been carried out using antibodies labelled with fluorescein (figure 5.14), radioiodine (figure 5.15) and peroxidase (figure 5.13), and indirectly with ferritin as described in the preceding section.

AGGLUTINATION

Whereas the cross-linking of multivalent protein antigens by antibody leads to precipitation, cross-linking of cells or large particles by antibody directed against surface antigens leads to agglutination. Since most cells are electrically charged, a reasonable number of antibody links between two cells is

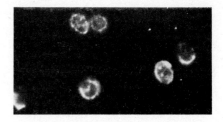

FIGURE 5.14. Antigens on the surface of viable human thyroid cells as demonstrated with thyroid autoantibodies in the indirect test. Note the patchy distribution. (Courtesy of Mrs. H. Lindqvist; after Fagreus A. & Jonsson J.)

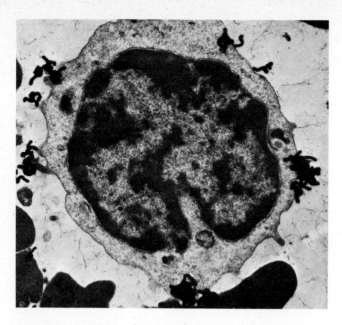

FIGURE 5.15. Electron microscopic autoradiograph of rabbit lymphocyte treated with ^{125}I-labelled antiallotype antibodies showing binding of the radioactive isoantibody to immunoglobulin determinants (probably antigen receptors) on the cell surface. Decay of an isotopic atom releases an electron which produces a track in the photographic emulsion. (Courtesy of Dr. G. Jones and Miss V. Petts.)

required before the mutual repulsion is overcome. Thus agglutination of cells bearing only a small number of determinants may be difficult to achieve unless special methods such as treatment with an antiglobulin reagent are used. Similarly, the higher avidity of multivalent IgM antibody relative to IgG (cf. p. 91) makes the former more effective as an agglutinating agent, molecule for molecule.

Agglutination reactions are used to identify bacteria and to type red cells; they have been observed with leucocytes and platelets and even with spermatozoa in certain cases of male infertility due to sperm agglutinins. Because of its sensitivity and convenience, the test has been extended to the identification of antibodies to soluble antigens which have been artificially coated onto various types of particle. Red cells have been popular and they can be coated with proteins after first modifying their surface with tannic acid or chromium chloride, or by direct use of bifunctional cross-linking agents such as bis-diazobenzidine. The tests are usually carried out in the wells of plastic agglutination trays where the settling pattern of the cells

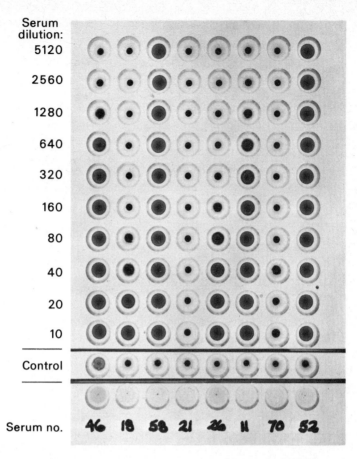

Serum dilution:
5120
2560
1280
640
320
160
80
40
20
10
Control
Serum no.   46   18   58   21   26   11   70   52

FIGURE 5.16. Tanned red cell haemagglutination test for thyroglobulin autoantibodies. Thyroglobulin-coated cells were added to dilutions of patients' sera. Uncoated cells were added to a 1:10 dilution of serum as a control. In a positive reaction, the cells settle as a carpet over the bottom of the cup. Because of the 'V'-shaped cross-section of these cups, in negative reactions the cells fall into the base of the 'V' forming a small easily recognizable button. The reciprocal of the highest serum dilution giving an unequivocally positive reaction is termed the *titre*. The titres reading from left to right are: 640, 20, > 5,120, neg, 40, 320, neg, > 5,120. The control for serum No. 46 was slightly positive and this serum should be tested again after absorption with uncoated cells.

on the bottom of the cup may be observed (figure 5.16); this provides a more sensitive indicator than macroscopic clumping. Inert particles such as bentonite and polystyrene latex have also been coated with antigens for agglutination reactions particularly those used to detect the rheumatoid factors (figure 5.17).

When two different cell types which share a common surface

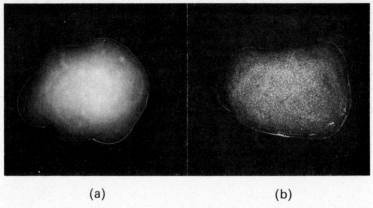

(a)   (b)

FIGURE 5.17. Macroscopic agglutination of latex coated with human IgG by serum from a patient with rheumatoid arthritis. This contains rheumatoid factor, an autoantibody directed against determinants on slightly altered IgG exposed by coating onto the latex surface. (a) normal serum, (b) patient's serum.

antigen are mixed in the presence of antibody, a 'mixed agglutination' reaction is seen. By this means the presence of the Group A antigen could be demonstrated on the surface of certain human cell lines in culture since they gave a mixed agglutinate with group A erythrocytes on addition of anti-A.

OPSONIC ADHERENCE

On combination with antigen, IgG antibodies develop an increased binding affinity for specific sites on the surface of polymorphonuclear leucocytes and macrophages. To take one example, bacteria coated with antibody become 'opsonized'— i.e. 'ready for the table' or 'tasty for the phagocytes'—and will adhere to phagocytic cells; this in turn facilitates the engulfment and subsequent digestion of the micro-organisms. Opsonic adherence and the related *immune adherence* reactions which involve binding through complement components (see below) are of major importance in the defence against infection. They may also be concerned in the removal of lymphocytes from the circulation by anti-lymphocyte serum and of red cells by the autoantibodies in autoimmune haemolytic anaemia. Immune complexes formed with soluble antigens will also adhere to phagocytic cells.

STIMULATION

A quite unexpected phenomenon has been observed in that antibodies to cell-surface components may sometimes lead not

116

to cytotoxic reactions as discussed below, but to actual stimulation of the cell. This probably occurs if the antibodies are directed against receptors on the surface which can generate a stimulatory signal when triggered by combination with the antibody. Examples are:

(i) The transformation and mitosis induced in small lymphocytes by anti-lymphocyte serum and anti-immunoglobulin sera *in vitro*. The latter combine with the immunoglobulin-like antigen receptors on the cell surface and mimic the configurational changes produced by antigen which activate the cell.

(ii) Degranulation of human mast cells by anti-IgE serum. The anti-IgE brings about the same sequence of changes as would specific antigen combining with the surface bound IgE molecules.

(iii) Stimulation of thyroid cells by autoantibodies present in the serum of patients with thyrotoxicosis (long acting thyroid stimulator, chapter 9).

(iv) Parthenogenetic division of sea-urchin eggs by antibody.

Stimulation may also be observed at the molecular level as in the increase in enzymic activity of certain penicillinase and β-galactosidase variants caused by addition of the appropriate antibodies which induce allosteric changes in the enzyme conformation.

CYTOTOXIC REACTIONS

If antibodies directed against the surface of cells are able to fix certain components present in the extracellular fluids, collectively termed *complement*, a cytotoxic reaction may occur. Historically, complement activity was recognized by Bordet who showed that the lytic activity against red cells of freshly drawn rabbit-sheep erythrocyte serum was lost on ageing or heating to 56°C for half-an-hour but could be restored by addition of fresh serum from an unimmunized rabbit. Thus, for haemolysis one requires a relatively heat stable factor, the antibody, plus a heat labile factor, complement, present in all fresh sera.

Complement

NATURE OF COMPLEMENT

The classical activity ascribed to complement (C') depends upon the operation of nine protein components (C1–C9) acting in sequence of which the first consists of three major subfractions termed C1q, C1r and C1s. Some of the characteristics of the three most abundant components are given in table 5.1:

TABLE 5.1.

	C1q	C4	C3
Serum concn., μg/ml	100–200	400	1,200
Molecular weight	400,000	230,000	185,000
Thermolability	+	–	–
Immunoelectrophoresis		β_{1E}	β_{1C}

When the first component is activated by an immune complex (e.g. antibody bound to a red cell), it acquires the ability to activate several molecules of the next component in the sequence; each of these is then able to act upon the next component and so on producing a cascade effect with amplification. In this way, the triggering of one molecule of C1 can lead to the activation of thousands of the later components. At each stage, activation is accompanied by the appearance of a new enzymic activity and since one enzyme molecule can process several substrate molecules, so each complement factor can cause the processing or activation of many molecules of the next component in the sequence (figure 5.18). The terminal components of the complement cascade have the ability to punch a 'functional hole' through the cell membrane on which they are fixed, perhaps through transformation into an active phospholipase, and this leads to cell death. Thus, through this sequential amplification process, the activation of one C1 molecule can lead to a macroscopic event, namely the lysis of a cell. As will be seen later, the intermediate stages in the complement sequence also

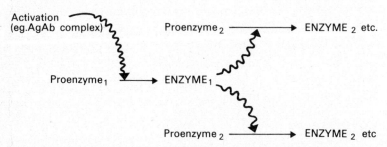

FIGURE 5.18. Enzymic basis of the amplifying complement cascade. The activated *enzyme₁* splits a peptide fragment from several molecules of *proenzyme₂* which all become active *enzyme₂* molecules capable of splitting *proenzyme₃* and so on.

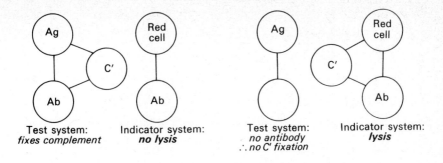

FIGURE 5.19. Complement fixation test. Antigen and antibody are
incubated in the presence of guinea-pig serum which acts as a source of
complement. Then the indicator system consisting of sheep red cells coated
with antibody is added.

(a) When antigen and antibody are present in the test system they fix
complement and none remains to lyse the added indicator system.

(b) When antigen or antibody is lacking in the test system, complement
is available to lyse the sensitized indicator cells.

give rise to other biological activities which are of importance in
health and disease. Like the blood clotting system, the complement components have a complex of inhibitors to regulate
activation.

THE COMPLEMENT FIXATION TEST (CFT)

The ability of certain immune complexes to bind or 'fix' the
components of complement may be used as a test for antibodies
if one has a known antigen and *vice versa*. To detect the consumption of complement by the test system, indicator cells
consisting of red cells coated with antibody are then added
(figure 5.19). Complement is measured as an activity as are
other enzyme systems and is expressed in terms of the degree of
lysis of a standard suspension of optimally coated sheep red
cells produced within a fixed time (figure 5.20).

The CFT is used routinely for diagnostic purposes as for
example the Wasserman reaction for syphilis and the CF reaction for 'Australia antigen' associated with one of the hepatitis viruses. Many of the autoantibodies to insoluble sub-
cellular components are detected by the CFT and in general it
is a convenient test for studying this type of antigen.

ACTIVATION OF COMPLEMENT

The activation of C1 is initiated by binding through C1q to C_{H2}
sites on the immunoglobulins forming a complex with antigen.

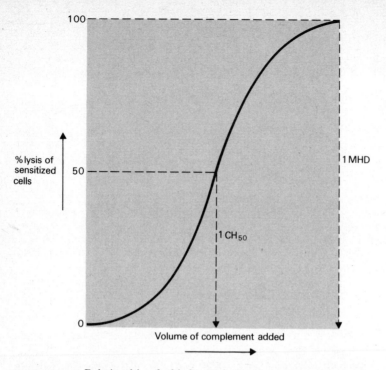

FIGURE 5.20. Relationship of added complement to percentage lysis of standard suspension of sensitized red cells. At the 50 per cent lysis point, the curve is steep and the amount of C' giving 50 per cent lysis (1 CH_{50}) can be accurately determined. The curve only gradually reaches 100 per cent lysis and the amount of C' giving 100 per cent lysis (1 Minimum Haemolytic Dose: 1 MHD) is less precisely assessed. The MHD is nonetheless adequate for routine serological purposes but for more accurate work the CH_{50} unit is preferred.

Aggregation of immunoglobulin as by heating to 60°C for 20 minutes also leads to the changes in structure which allow complement binding. Different immunoglobulin classes have different Fc structures and only IgG and IgM can bind C1. There are differences even within the IgG subclasses: IgG1 and IgG3 fix complement well, IgG2 modestly and IgG4 poorly, if at all. C1q is polyvalent with respect to Ig binding and consists of a central core surrounded by 6 identical subunits disposed at the corners of a regular octahedron. At least two of these subunits must bind to immunoglobulin $C_{H}2$ sites for activation of C1q. With IgM this is less of a problem since several Fc regions are available within a single molecule, but IgG antibodies will only fix complement when two or more molecules are bound to closely adjacent sites on the antigen. It is for this reason that IgM antibodies to red cells have a high haemolytic efficiency

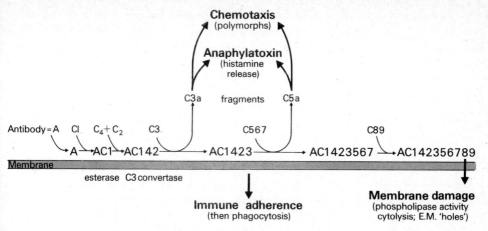

FIGURE 5.21. Sequence of complement activation showing formation of fragments chemotactic for polymorphs and with anaphylatoxin activity causing histamine release. Activated C567 complex is also chemotactic. Immune adherence through C3 to macrophages, platelets or red cells facilitates phagocytosis. Fixation of C8 and 9 generates cytolytic activity. Cells bearing AC1423567 are susceptible to cytotoxic attack by lymphocytes.

since a 'single hit' will produce full complement activation and cell death. With IgG antibodies, a far larger number of 'hits' will be required before, by chance, two IgG antibodies are bound at adjacent sites and are then able to initiate the complement sequence.

Complement can be activated by another route, the so-called *alternate pathway* (see below). This can be stimulated by certain cell wall polysaccharides such as bacterial endotoxin and yeast zymosan, by some aggregated immunoglobulins such as human IgA and guinea pig IgG1 known to be ineffective for C1q binding, and, as we shall see later, by a feedback mechanism from the classical pathway.

THE COMPLEMENT SEQUENCE (figure 5.21)

Classical pathway

C1q is linked in a trimolecular complex, possibly through calcium to C1r and C1s. After the binding of C1q to the Fc regions of an immune complex, C1s acquires esterase activity and brings about the activation and transfer to hydrophobic sites on the membrane (or immune complex) of first C4 and then C2 (unfortunately components were numbered before the sequence was established). This complex has 'C3-convertase' activity and acts upon C3 in solution with two main results:

1. Fragments (C3a) are released which are *chemotactic* for poly-morphonuclear leucocytes and which have *anaphylatoxin* activity in that they cause histamine release presumably from mast cells.

2. A very large number of modified C3 molecules (C3b) are transferred to the surface membrane. There are specific binding sites for the modified C3 on macrophages (all mammalian species studied), platelets (rabbits) and red cells (primates) which allow *immune adherence* of the antigen–antibody-C3 complex to these cells so facilitating subsequent phagocytosis (figure 5.21). Furthermore, after inactivation by KAF (con-glutinogen-activating factor), the bound C3 presents a new structural configuration not present on the native molecule which can provoke the formation of the autoantibody *immuno-conglutinin*.

Alternate pathway

In the classical pathway we have just discussed, the active C3b fragment is formed by the action of a C142 convertase. Another convertase, the C3 activator (C3A) can be generated by a distinct series of reactions collectively termed the alternate pathway. C3A is derived from a precursor (C3PA) by the action of a magnesium dependent enzyme, C3PAse, which itself can be formed in two ways (figure 5.22). The first involves activation of properdin by extrinsic agents such as endotoxin or aggregated IgA, and the second, positive feedback through C3b, i.e. the product of C3 cleavage catalyses the reaction which leads to a greater activation of C3A. This loop in the complement chain is modulated by the C3 inactivator KAF which destroys the haemolytic and immune adherence re-activity of C3b and renders it susceptible to attack by trypsin-like enzymes. Whenever C3b is generated by the classical C1 pathway it might be expected to activate the alternate pathway through this feedback mechanism.

Post C3 pathway

The complement sequence reaches its full amplitude at the C3 stage. Thereafter C5 is split to give a C5a fragment with che-motactic and anaphylatoxin activity while the C5b binds as a complex with C6 and 7 to form a thermostable site on the membrane. Finally the terminal components C8 and C9 are bound and these generate *membrane damage* through phospho-

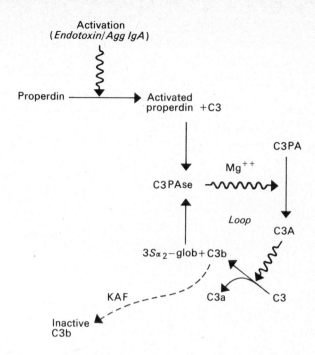

FIGURE 5.22. The alternate complement pathway for activation of C3. ⁓⁓⁓⟶ represents activation of the reaction indicated by the straight arrow ⟶ .

C3A = C3 activator or convertase (synonym GGG); C3PA = C3 proactivator or C3A precursor (≡GBG); C3PAse = C3PA activating enzyme (≡GBGase); KAF = conglutinogen activating factor.

lipase-like activity. The cytolytic component is C8 but C9 enhances its activity (figure 5.21).

Yet more complexity is introduced by the phenomenon of *reactive lysis* (Lachmann & Thomson); a proportion of the activated C5b67 complexes formed remain free and not only are they chemotactic for neutrophils but are also able to bind to 'innocent' cells in the vicinity. Once fixed to the cell surface they can complete the complement sequence by binding C8, 9 with resultant cell lysis.

There is evidence that the C′ sequence can sometimes be short-circuited as for example in the activation of membrane C8 in normal lymphoid cells which can be shown to be cytotoxic for chicken erythrocytes coated with C1–7.

ROLE IN DEFENCE

Cytolysis

The full complement system leading to membrane damage can cause bacteriolysis in Gram-negative organisms by allowing

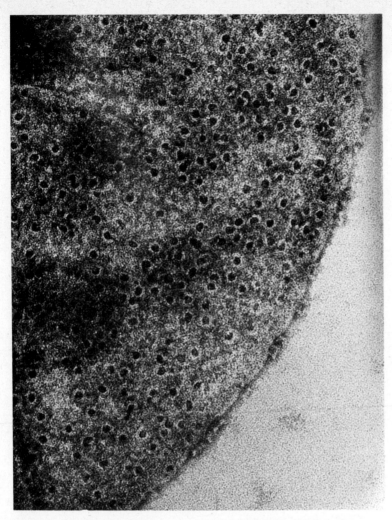

FIGURE 5.23. Multiple lesions in cell wall of *Escherichia coli* bacterium caused by interaction with IgM antibody and complement. Each lesion is caused by a single IgM molecule and shows as a 'dark pit' due to penetration by the 'negative stain'. Magnification ×400,000. (Courtesy of Drs. R. Dourmashkin and J.H. Humphrey.)

lysozyme to reach the plasma membrane where it destroys the mucopeptide layer. Negatively stained preparations in the electron microscope show the 'pits' on the surface (figure 5.23) which correspond with individual sites of complement activation and which resemble those seen on the red cell.

Immune adherence

This is probably a major pathway leading to phagocytosis of micro-organisms after coating with opsonizing antibody and C′

or after activation of the alternative complement pathway. Since many C3 molecules are bound onto the surface at each site of C' activation, adherence to macrophages and polymorphs will occur more frequently through C3 than IgG binding.

Immunoconglutinin

This may play a role by agglutinating relatively small complexes containing bound C3 thereby making them more susceptible to phagocytosis.

Inflammation

The fragments produced during complement consumption stimulate two helpful features of the acute inflammatory response. First, the chemotactic factors attract phagocytic neutrophil polymorphs to the site of C' activation, and secondly anaphylatoxin, through histamine release, increases vascular permeability and hence the flow of serum antibody and more C' to the infected area.

ROLE IN DISEASE

Complement is implicated in disease processes involving cytotoxic and immune-complex mediated hypersensitivities which will be discussed in more detail in the following chapter. Cytotoxic reactions are seen in nephrotoxic nephritis and autoimmune haemolytic anaemia. Complexes formed in antibody excess giving rise to immune vasculitis of the Arthus type are seen, for example, in Farmer's lung and cryoglobulinaemia with cutaneous vasculitis; soluble complexes formed in antigen excess give 'serum sickness' type reactions with considerable deposition in the kidney glomeruli as found in many forms of chronic glomerulonephritis.

Endotoxin shock in rabbits is a complex phenomenon in which the alternate pathway becomes activated. Endotoxin coated with C3 sticks to platelets by immune adherence and C567 complexes generated cause platelet destruction by reactive lysis with release of clotting factor III.

COMPLEMENT DEFICIENCIES

A transient fall in C' can be induced by injection of aggregated IgG or of a cobra venom enzyme which inhibits the activation of C3, but this state is difficult to maintain. Permanent deficiencies in certain components have been observed though. Some strains of mice completely lack C5 and rabbits with an absolute deficiency of C6 have been bred. These animals are not particularly susceptible to infection and it would appear that the full operation of the C' system up to C8,9 is not essential for survival; adequate protection must be afforded by opsonizing antibodies and the immune adherence mechanism.

In man a few cases with relative deficiency of C2 have been identified but the amounts present do not seem to limit the overall rate of C' activation. An inhibitor of active C1 is lacking in hereditary angioneurotic oedema and this can lead to recurring episodes of acute circumscribed non-inflammatory oedema. The importance of C' in defence against infection is emphasized by the occurrence of repeated infections in a patient lacking KAF. Because of his inability to destroy C3b there is continual activation of the alternate pathway through the feedback loop leading to very low C3 and C3PA levels with normal C1, 4 and 2.

Neutralization of biological activity

To continue our discussion on the interaction of antigen and antibody *in vitro*, we may focus attention on a number of biological reactions which can be inhibited by addition of specific antibody. Thus the agglutination of red cells by interaction of influenza virus with receptors on the erythrocyte surface can be blocked by antiviral antibodies and this forms the basis for their serological detection. A test for antibodies to salmonella H antigen present on the flagella depends upon their ability to inhibit the motility of the bacteria *in vitro*. Likewise, mycoplasma antibodies can be demonstrated by their inhibitory effect on the metabolism of the organisms in culture. Antibodies to hormones such as insulin and TSH can be used to probe the specificity of biological reactions *in vitro*; for example the specificity of the insulin-like activity of a serum sample on rat epididymal fat pad can be checked by the neutralizing effect of an antiserum. This type of approach will clearly have many applications.

Further reading

Clausen J. (1969) *Immunochemical techniques for the identification and estimation of macromolecules.* North-Holland, Amsterdam.
Holborow E.J. (ed.) (1970) *Standardization in Immunofluorescence.* Blackwell Scientific Publications, Oxford.

Hudson L. & Hay F.C. (1974) *Practical Immunology*. Blackwell Scientific Publications, Oxford.

Lachmann P.J. & Nicol P. (1973) Reaction mechanism of the alternative pathway of complement fixation. *Lancet*, **1**, 465.

Müller-Eberhard H.J. (1968) Chemistry and reaction mechanisms of complement. *Adv.Immunol.*, Vol. 8.

Roitt I.M. & Doniach D. (1973) *Manual on Autoimmune Serology*. (Obtainable from Immunology Division, W.H.O., Geneva.)

Ruddy S., Gigli I. & Austen K.F. (1972) The complement system of man. *N.Engl.J.Med.*, **287**, 489, 545, 592 & 642.

Weir D.M. (ed.) (1973) *Handbook of Experimental Immunology*, 2nd ed. Blackwell Scientific Publications, Oxford.

Williams C.A. & Chase M.W. (1967–71) *Methods in Immunology and Immunochemistry*, Vols. I–IV. Academic Press, London.

6 Hypersensitivity

When an individual has been immunologically primed or sensitized, further contact with antigen can lead not only to secondary boosting of the immune response but can also cause tissue-damaging reactions. We speak of *hypersensitivity reactions* and a state of *hypersensitivity*. Coombs and Gell defined four types of hypersensitivity, to which can be added a fifth, viz. 'stimulatory', which they mention. Types I, II, III and V depend on the interaction of antigen with humoral antibody and tend to be called 'immediate' type reactions although some are more immediate than others! Type IV involves receptors bound to the lymphocyte surface and because of the longer time course this has in the past been referred to as 'delayed-type sensitivity'. The essential basis of these reactions are summarized below and then each considered separately in more detail.

TYPE I—ANAPHYLACTIC-TYPE SENSITIVITY

The antigen reacts with a specific class of antibody bound to mast cells or circulating basophils through a specialized region of the Fc piece. This leads to degranulation of the mast cells and release of vasoactive amines (figure 6.1). These antibodies are termed homocytotropic (also referred to as reagins).

TYPE II—CYTOTOXIC-TYPE HYPERSENSITIVITY

Antibodies binding to an antigen on the cell surface cause (i) phagocytosis of the cell through opsonic (Fc) or immune (C3) adherence, (ii) non-phagocytic extracellular cytotoxicity by killer (K) cells with receptors for IgFc and (iii) lysis through the operation of the full complement system up to C8, 9 (figure 6.2).

TYPE III—COMPLEX-MEDIATED HYPERSENSITIVITY

The formation of complexes between antigen and humoral antibody can lead to activation of the complement system and to

129

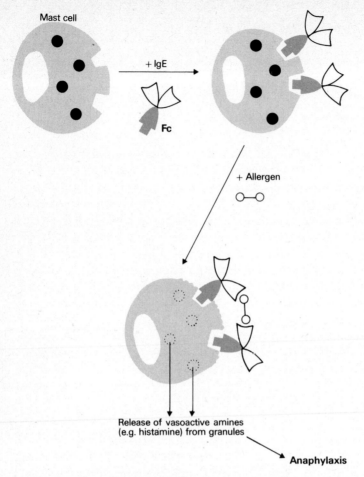

FIGURE 6.1. Type I—Anaphylactic-type hypersensitivity. Mast-cell degranulation following interaction of antigen with bound homocytotropic (reaginic) antibodies. Slow reacting substance A (SRS-A) is released during anaphylaxis, but its origin is unknown.

the aggregation of platelets with the consequences listed in figure 6.3.

TYPE IV—CELL-MEDIATED (DELAYED-TYPE) HYPERSENSITIVITY

Thymic derived T-lymphocytes bearing specific receptors on their surface are stimulated by contact with antigen to release factors (termed 'lymphokines' by Dumonde) which mediate delayed-type hypersensitivity (e.g. Mantoux test for tuberculin sensitivity); in the reaction against tissue transplants, the stimulated lymphocytes transform into blast-like cells capable of

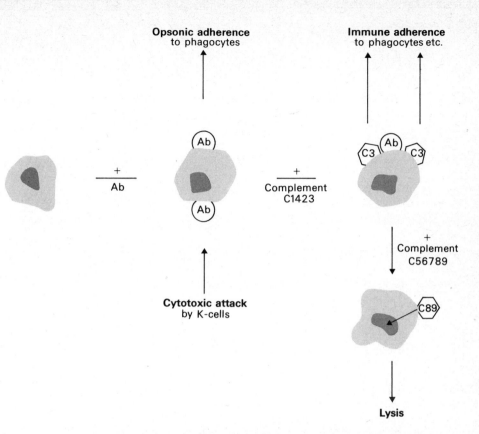

Opsonic adherence
to phagocytes

Immune adherence
to phagocytes etc.

Ab

+
Ab

+
Complement
C1423

C3 Ab C3

+
Complement
C56789

Cytotoxic attack
by K-cells

C89

Lysis

FIGURE 6.2 Type II—Cytotoxic-type hypersensitivity. Antibodies
directed against cell surface antigens cause cell death not only by
C-dependent lysis but also by adherence reactions leading to phagocytosis
or through non-phagocytic extracellular killing by certain lymphoreticular
cells (K-cell activity).

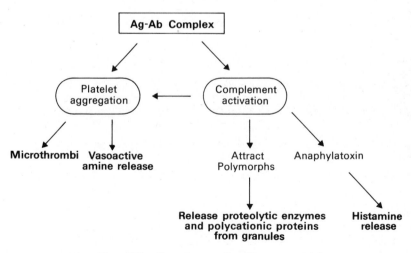

Ag-Ab Complex

Platelet
aggregation

Complement
activation

Microthrombi **Vasoactive
amine release**

Attract
Polymorphs

Anaphylatoxin

**Release proteolytic enzymes
and polycationic proteins
from granules**

**Histamine
release**

FIGURE 6.3. Type III—Complex-mediated hypersensitivity.

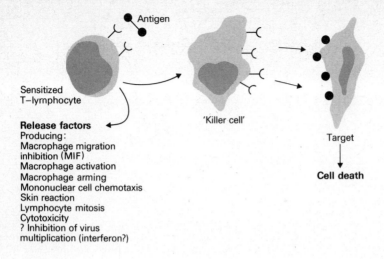

Antigen

Sensitized
T–lymphocyte

'Killer cell'

Release factors
Producing:
Macrophage migration
inhibition (MIF)
Macrophage activation
Macrophage arming
Mononuclear cell chemotaxis
Skin reaction
Lymphocyte mitosis
Cytotoxicity
? Inhibition of virus
multiplication (interferon?)

Target

Cell death

FIGURE 6.4. Type IV—Cell-mediated (delayed-type) hypersensitivity.

killing target cells bearing the histocompatibility antigens of the graft (figure 6.4).

TYPE V—STIMULATORY HYPERSENSITIVITY

Non-complement fixing antibodies directed against certain cell surface components may actually stimulate rather than destroy the cell (figure 6.5). Theoretically stimulation could also occur through the development of antibodies to naturally occurring mitotic inhibitors in the circulation.

Type I—Anaphylactic-type sensitivity

SYSTEMIC ANAPHYLAXIS

A single injection of 1 mg of an antigen such as egg albumin into a guinea-pig has no obvious effect. However, if the injection is repeated two to three weeks later, the sensitized animal reacts very dramatically with the symptoms of generalized anaphylaxis; almost immediately the guinea-pig begins to wheeze and within a few minutes dies from asphyxia. Examination shows intense constriction of the bronchioles and bronchi and generally there is (a) contraction of smooth muscle and (b) dilatation of capillaries.

Similar reactions can occur in human subjects and have been

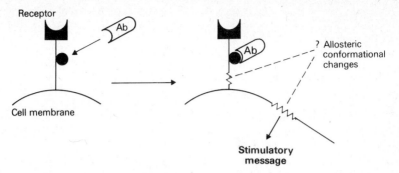

Receptor

Ab

? Allosteric
conformational
changes

Cell membrane

Stimulatory
message

FIGURE 6.5. Type V—Stimulatory hypersensitivity.

observed following insect bites or injections of penicillin in appropriately sensitive individuals. In many instances only a timely intravenous injection of adrenaline to counter the smooth muscle contraction and capillary dilatation can prevent death.

MECHANISM OF ANAPHYLAXIS

Sir Henry Dale recognized that histamine mimics the systemic changes of anaphylaxis and furthermore that the uterus from a sensitized guinea-pig releases histamine and contracts on exposure to antigen (Schultz–Dale technique). Serum from such an animal can passively sensitize the uterus from a normal guinea-pig so that it, too, will contract on addition of the specific antigen. Contraction is associated with an explosive degranulation of the mast cells which is responsible for the release of histamine and, in certain species, of another mediator of anaphylaxis, 5-hydroxytryptamine (serotonin). A third mediator, slow reacting substance (SRS-A) capable of inducing a prolonged contraction of certain smooth muscles is also released but its origin in the tissue is unknown.

It seems clear that the mast cells become coated by a particular type of antibody whose Fc region can bind specifically to sites on the mast cell surface. The most effective homocytotropic antibodies belong to the IgE class but it is clear that IgG antibodies can also act as reagins although the extent of their contribution to the allergic state in the human is not yet resolved. IgG reagins differ from IgE in their relative insensitivity to mild heat and 2-mercaptoethanol reduction and especially in their lower binding affinity for mast cells; whereas IgE antibodies can be detected at the site of an intradermal injection into a normal individual for several weeks, IgG disperses within a day or so. The technique of *passive cutaneous anaphylaxis* (PCA) introduced by Ovary utilizes this dermal reaction as a highly sensitive indicator for reaginic antibodies. For example, high dilutions of guinea-pig serum containing γ_1-globulin antibodies may be injected into the skin of a normal animal and following the intravenous injection of antigen with a dye such as Evans' Blue, the anaphylactic reaction in the skin will lead to release of vasoactive amines and hence a local 'blueing'.

Degranulation of the mast cell occurs when the bound homocytotropic antibodies are cross-linked either by specific antigen (figure 6.1) or by the corresponding divalent anti-immunoglobulin (e.g. anti-IgE or anti-light chain); univalent (Fab) anti-IgE will not cause degranulation. This cross-linking reaction must induce a membrane signal linked in some way with the adenyl cyclase system since it is known that the maintenance of intracellular cyclic-AMP concentrations is probably required for stability of the mast-cell granules and agents which act to increase these levels tend to inhibit anaphylaxis.

ATOPIC ALLERGY

Nearly 10 per cent of the population suffer to a greater or lesser degree with allergies involving localized anaphylactic reactions to extrinsic allergens such as grass pollens, animal danders, mites in house dust and so on. Contact of the allergen with cell-bound IgE in the bronchial tree, the nasal mucosa and the conjunctival tissues releases mediators of anaphylaxis and produces the symptoms of asthma or hay fever as the case may be. For those unfortunates sensitized to foods such as the strawberry, the price of indulgence may be a generalized urticaria caused by reaction in the skin to materials absorbed from the gut into the blood stream. Acute anaphylaxis although rare may occur in highly sensitive subjects after an insect bite or injections of penicillin or procaine.

Sensitivity is normally assessed by the response to intradermal challenge with antigen. The release of histamine and other mediators rapidly produces a wheal and erythema (figure 6.10a), maximal within 30 minutes and then subsiding. The responsible IgE antibodies can be demonstrated by the ability of patient's serum to passively sensitize the skin of normal humans (Praüsnitz–Kustner or 'P–K' test) or preferably of monkeys. This passive sensitization of human skin can be blocked most effectively by prior injection of a myeloma of IgE rather than of any other class. The interpretation is that the specialized sites on the skin mast cells become fully saturated by binding to the Fc regions of the IgE myeloma globulin which blocks the subsequent attachment of specific IgE antibodies.

The lymphocytes from patients with atopic allergy undergo blast-cell transformation and release a migration inhibition factor on contact with allergen. These are thought to be indicators of cell-mediated immunity, and delayed-type hypersensitivity reactions (see below) have been elicited in some patients in whom the immediate response had been suppressed with anti-histamines. The reactive T-lymphocytes giving rise to these phenomena might also function as helper cells co-operating in the synthesis of IgE antibodies by B-cells.

The symptoms of atopic allergy are largely but not always completely controllable by anti-histamines. Other effective drugs such as Isoprenaline and disodium cromoglycate (Intal) probably act by stabilizing the adenyl cyclase–cyclic-AMP system to prevent vasoactive amine release. Attempts to desensitize patients immunologically by repeated treatment with allergen have at least the merit of a long history and in a significant but as yet unpredictable proportion of patients can lead to worthwhile improvement. It has generally been assumed that the purpose of these inoculations was to boost the synthesis of 'blocking' IgG antibody whose function was to divert the allergen from contact with tissue-bound IgE. However, if T-lymphocyte co-operation is important for IgE synthesis, the beneficial effects of antigen injection may also be mediated through induction of tolerance in the appropriate T-cells. Better results must ultimately be attainable when we understand the rationale of 'hyposensitization' through the use of purified allergens, assessment of T-cell reactivity and quantitative measurement of specific IgG, IgA and IgE antibodies in individuals undergoing treatment. The affinity of these antibodies and their availability at local sites of allergen challenge such as the nasal mucosa are factors which cannot be ignored.

There is a strong familial predisposition to the development of these disorders but although this is linked to inheritance of a given HL-A haplotype within any one family, no association with specific HL-A types has so far come to light. Curiously, it is said that patients with allergy are less likely than their non-atopic counterparts to develop tumours.

Type II—Cytotoxic-type hypersensitivity

Where an antigen is present on the surface of a cell, combination with antibody will encourage the demise of that cell by promot-

135

ing contact with phagocytes either by reduction in surface charge, by opsonic adherence directly through the Fc or by immune adherence through bound C3. Cell death may also occur through activation of the full complement system up to C8 and C9 producing direct membrane damage. Although in the case of haemolytic antibodies, the generation of a single active complement site is enough to cause erythrocyte lysis, other cells appear to have repair mechanisms and it is likely that several complement sites need to be recruited in order to overwhelm the cell's defences.

The operation of a quite distinct cytotoxic mechanism is suggested by Perlmann's finding that target cells coated with IgG antibody in culture can be killed 'non-specifically' through an extracellular non-phagocytic mechanism involving non-sensitized lymphoreticular cells which bind to the target by their specific receptors for IgG Fc (figure 6.6). This so-called 'K-cell activity' may be exhibited by typical phagocytic macrophages but even when the phagocytic cells have been removed from a white cell suspension prepared from blood, lymphoid tissue or bone-marrow, considerable K-cell activity remains. It has been established that these non-phagocytic K-cells are neither T- nor Ig-bearing B-lymphocytes. In the mouse they show certain similarities to cells of the myeloid series in that they are glass adherent and inhibited by aggregated IgG subclasses known to block the Fc receptors on monocytes. A proportion of K-cells in the human do seem to have rather different characteristics in terms of adherence and subclass inhibition but although they bear some morphological resemblance to lymphocytes there is at present no other evidence to link them with this family of cells. In all likelihood a number of different cell types will eventually prove to have

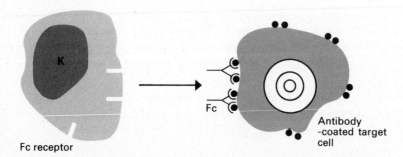

FIGURE 6.6. Killing of antibody-coated target by K-cell. The surface receptors for Ig Fc region bind the K-cell to the target which is then killed by an extracellular mechanism. Several different cell types may display K-cell activity.

K-activity. Functionally, this extra-cellular cytotoxic mechanism would be expected to be of significance where the target is too large for ingestion by phagocytosis e.g. large parasites and solid tumours. Evidence to be discussed later in Chapter 8 would favour a role in some forms of tumour immunity when K cells could acquire specific cytotoxic activity by arming with immune complexes (cf. figure 8.10).

ISOIMMUNE REACTIONS

Transfusion reactions

Individuals normally possess antibodies to antigens of the ABO blood group system not present on their own erythrocytes. A person of blood group A will possess anti-B and so on. These *isohaemagglutinins* are usually IgM and are thought to arise through immunization against antigens of the gut flora which are similar to the blood group substances so that the antibodies formed cross-react with the appropriate red cell type. If an individual is blood group A, he will be tolerant to antigens closely similar to A and will only form cross-reacting antibodies capable of agglutinating B red cells; similarly an O individual will make anti-A and anti-B. On transfusion, mismatched red cells will be coated by the isohaemagglutinins and cause severe reactions.

Rhesus incompatibility

A mother with an Rh negative blood group can readily be sensitized by red cells from a baby carrying Rh antigens (usually the D-antigen). This occurs most often at the birth of the first child when a placental bleed can release a large number of the baby's erythrocytes into the mother. The antibodies formed are predominantly of the IgG class and are able to cross the placenta in any subsequent pregnancy. Reaction with the D-antigen on the foetal red cells leads to their destruction through opsonic adherence giving haemolytic disease of the newborn (figure 6.7).

These anti-D antibodies fail to agglutinate RhD + red cells *in vitro* and have therefore been termed 'incomplete'. Erythrocytes coated with anti-D can be made to agglutinate by addition of albumin or of an anti-immunoglobulin serum (Coombs' reagent). Two factors are probably responsible for these phenomena: the high negative charge on the erythrocyte surface and the relative sparsity of the D-sites. The small number of direct bridges that can be formed by D-antibodies

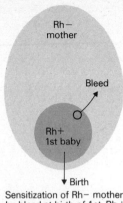
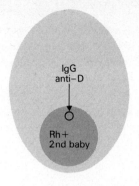

Rh−
mother

Bleed

Rh+
1st baby

Birth

Sensitization of Rh− mother
by bleed at birth of 1st Rh+
baby leading to synthesis of
anti−D.

IgG
anti−D

Rh+
2nd baby

D+ erythrocytes in 2nd child
affected by IgG anti−D crossing
the placenta.

FIGURE 6.7. Haemolytic disease of the newborn due to rhesus
incompatibility.

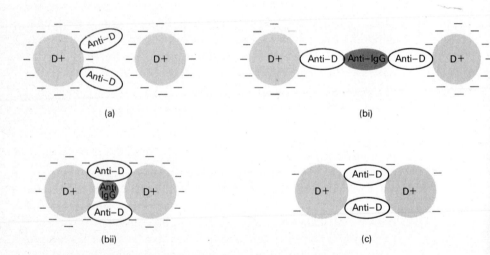

(a)

(bi)

(bii)

(c)

FIGURE 6.8. Agglutination of D red cells by incomplete anti-D in
presence of antiglobulin or albumin.

(a) No agglutination of Rh D + cells by anti-D in saline. Because of the
low density of D-antigen sites the few molecules of bound anti-D are
unable to overcome the repulsion of the negatively charged D+ red cells.

(b) Antiglobulin causes agglutination because (i) with an antiglobulin
bridge the cells are further apart and the repulsion less, and (ii) by cross-
linking (speculation this), the anti-D molecules effectively become
multivalent and thereby acquire a greatly increased avidity (cf. chapter 1,
p. 15).

(c) Albumin causes agglutination of cells coated with anti-D because it
modifies the surface charge and the repulsive forces are decreased.

138

between two red cells would have insufficient total binding energy to overcome the mutual repulsion of the erythrocytes (figure 6.8a). If an antiglobulin were added as an extra span in the 'bridge' the cells would not have to approach so closely and would not repel each other with such force (figure 6.8b(i)). Also, through cross-linking by the antiglobulin, the anti-D can become multivalent thereby greatly increasing its binding avidity (figure 6.8b(ii)). Alternatively, if albumin is added (or if the cells are treated with papain), the surface charge is modified and the bridging by anti-D alone is sufficient to agglutinate the cells (figure 6.8c).

If a mother has natural isohaemagglutinins which can react with any foetal erythrocytes reaching her circulation, sensitization to the D antigens is less likely due to 'deviation' of the red cells away from the antigen sensitive cells. For example, a group O Rh − ve mother with a group A Rh + ve baby would destroy any foetal erythrocytes with her anti-A before they could immunize to produce anti-D. In an extension of this principle, Rh − ve mothers are now treated prophylactically with small amounts of avid IgG anti-D at the time of birth of the first child, and this greatly reduces the risk of sensitization.

Organ transplants

A longstanding homograft which has withstood the first onslaught of the cell-mediated reaction can evoke humoral antibodies in the host directed against surface transplantation antigens on the graft. These may be directly cytotoxic, or cause adherence of phagocytic cells or 'non-specific' attack by K cells (cf. figure 6.2). They may also lead to platelet adherence when they combine with antigens on the surface of the vascular endothelium.

AUTOIMMUNE REACTIONS

Autoantibodies to the patient's own red cells are produced in autoimmune haemolytic anaemia. Red cells coated with these antibodies have a shortened half-life largely through their adherence to phagocytic cells. The serum of patients with Hashimoto's thyroiditis contain antibodies which in the presence of complement are directly cytotoxic for isolated human thyroid cells in culture. In Goodpasture's syndrome, antibodies to kidney glomerular basement membrane are present. Biopsies show these antibodies together with complement components bound to the basement membranes where the

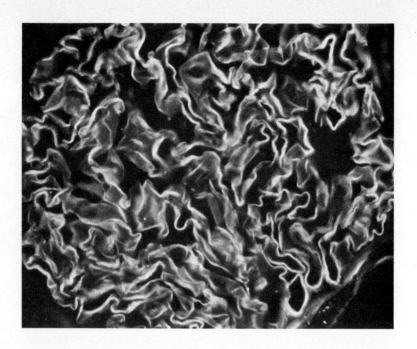

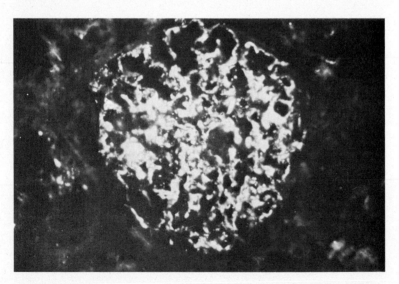

FIGURE 6.9. Glomerulonephritis: (a) due to linear deposition of antibody to glomerular basement membrane here visualized by staining the human kidney biopsy with a fluorescent anti-IgG (courtesy of Dr. F.J. Dixon) and (b) due to deposition of antigen–antibody complexes which can be seen as discrete masses lining the glomerular basement membrane following immunofluorescent staining with anti-IgG (courtesy of Dr. D. Doniach). Similar patterns to these are obtained with a fluorescent anti-β_{1C} (complement component C_3).

action of the full complement system leads to serious damage (figure 6.9a).

DRUG REACTIONS

Very complicated. Drugs may become coupled to body components and thereby undergo conversion from a hapten to a full antigen which will sensitize certain individuals (we don't know which). If IgE antibodies are produced, anaphylactic reactions can result. In some circumstances, particularly with topically applied ointments, cell-mediated hypersensitivity may be induced. In other cases where coupling to serum proteins occurs, the possibility of type III complex-mediated reactions may arise. In the present context we are concerned with those instances where the drug appears to form an antigenic complex with the surface of a formed element of the blood and evokes the production of antibodies which are cytotoxic for the cell-drug complex. When the drug is withdrawn, the sensitivity is no longer evident. Examples of this mechanism have been seen in the *haemolytic anaemia* sometimes associated with continued administration of chlorpromazine or phenacetin, in the *agranulocytosis* associated with the taking of amidopyrine or of quinidine, and the classic situation of *thrombocytopenic purpura* which may be produced by Sedormid. In the latter case, for instance, freshly drawn serum from the patient will lyse platelets in the presence but not in the absence of Sedormid; inactivation of complement by preheating the serum at $56°C$ for 30 minutes abrogates this effect.

Type III—Complex-mediated hypersensitivity

The union of soluble antigens and antibodies within the body may give rise to an acute inflammatory reaction (cf. figure 6.3). If complement is fixed, anaphylatoxins will be released as split products of C3 and C5 and these will cause histamine release with vascular permeability changes. The chemotactic factors also produced will lead to an influx of polymorphonuclear leucocytes which begin the phagocytosis of the immune complexes; this in turn results in the extracellular release from the polymorph granules of proteolytic enzymes (including neutral proteinases and collagenase), kinin-forming enzymes and polycationic proteins which increase vascular permeability through both mastocytolytic and histamine-independent mechanisms.

These will damage local tissues and intensify the inflammatory responses. Further damage may be mediated by reactive lysis (chapter 5, p. 123) in which activated C567 becomes attached to the surface of nearby cells and binds C8,9. Under appropriate conditions, platelets may be aggregated with two consequences: they provide yet a further source of vasoactive amines and may also form microthrombi which can lead to local ischaemia. (The discerning reader will appreciate the need for the complex system of inhibitors present in the body.)

The outcome of the formation of immune complexes *in vivo* depends not only on the absolute amounts of antigen and antibody, which determine the intensity of the reaction, but also on their *relative* proportions which govern the nature of the complexes (cf. precipitin curve, p. 5) and hence their distribution within the body. In gross *antibody excess* the complexes are rapidly precipitated and tend to be localized to the site of introduction of antigen whereas in *antigen excess*, soluble complexes are formed which may cause systemic reactions and be widely deposited in the kidneys, joints and skin.

ANTIBODY EXCESS (ARTHUS TYPE REACTIVITY)

Maurice Arthus found that injection of soluble antigen intradermally into hyperimmunized rabbits with high levels of precipitating antibody produced an erythematous and oedematous reaction (cf. figure 6.10b) reaching a peak at 3–8 hours and then usually resolving. The lesion was characterized by an intense infiltration with polymorphonuclear leukocytes (figure 6.11a). The injected antigen precipitates with antibody often within the venule and the complex binds complement; using the appropriate fluorescent reagents, antigen, immunoglobulin and complement components can all be demonstrated in this lesion. Anaphylatoxin is soon generated and causes histamine liberation. Local intravascular complexes will cause platelet aggregation and vasoactive amine release. This early phase is seen readily in man as an erythematous reaction which should not be confused with the immediate anaphylactic type I skin response. The formation of chemotactic factors leads to the influx of polymorphs and, as a result, erythema and oedema increase. The Arthus reaction can be blocked by depletion of complement or of the neutrophil polymorphs (by nitrogen mustard or specific anti-polymorph sera). There is evidence that an immediate anaphylactic type I response is mandatory for initiating the first stages of the Arthus reaction but whether

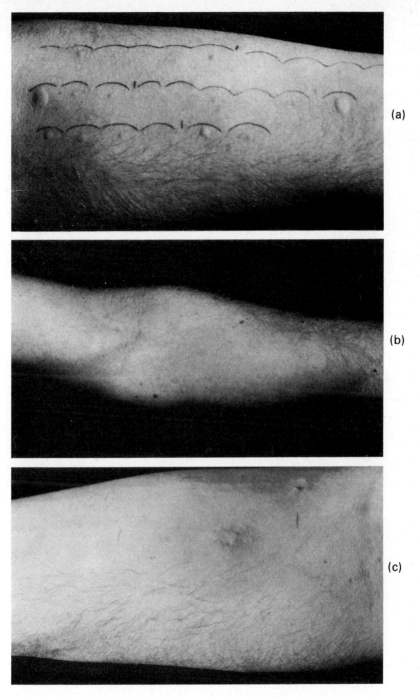

FIGURE 6.10. Comparison of intradermal reactions obtained in different forms of hypersensitivity: (a) Type I—anaphylactic: wheal and flare; (b) Type III—Arthus: erythema and oëdema; (c) Type IV—cell-mediated hypersensitivity: induration and erythema (courtesy of Prof. J. Pepys).

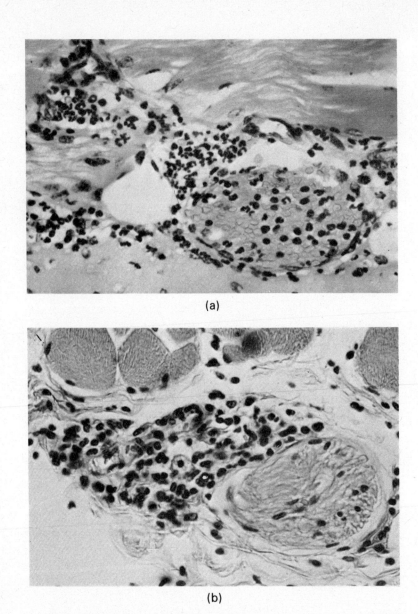

(a)

(b)

FIGURE 6.11. Histology of (a) Arthus and (b) cell-mediated hyper-sensitivity showing predominance of polymorphs and mononuclear cells respectively in the intradermal lesions. (Photographed from material kindly provided by Prof. J.L. Turk.)

this requires IgE or can be mediated by IgG reagins is uncertain.

Intrapulmonary Arthus-type reactions to inhaled antigen appear to be responsible for a number of hypersensitivity disorders in man. The severe respiratory difficulties associated with Farmer's lung occur within 6–8 hours of exposure to the dust from mouldy hay. The patients are found to be sensitized to thermophilic actinomycetes which grow in the mouldy hay and extracts of these organisms give precipitin reactions with the subject's serum and Arthus reactions on intradermal injection. Inhalation of bacterial spores present in dust from the hay introduces antigen into the lungs and a complex-mediated hypersensitivity reaction occurs. A similar situation arises in pigeon-fancier's disease where the antigen is probably serum protein present in the dust from dried faeces, and in many other cases where potentially antigenic materials are continually inhaled.

ANTIGEN EXCESS (SERUM SICKNESS)

Injection of relatively large doses of foreign serum (e.g. horse anti-diphtheria) used to be employed for various therapeutic purposes. It was not uncommon for a condition known as 'serum sickness' to arise some eight days after the injection. A rise in temperature, swollen lymph nodes, a generalized urticarial rash and painful swollen joints associated with a low serum complement and transient albuminuria could be encountered. These result from the deposition of soluble antigen–antibody complexes formed in antigen excess.

Some individuals begin to synthesize antibodies against the foreign protein—usually horse globulin. Since the antigen is still present in gross excess at that time (figure 6.12), soluble complexes of composition Ag_2Ab, Ag_3Ab_2, Ag_4Ab_3, etc. will be formed (cf. precipitin curve, figure 1.3, p. 5). The larger complexes can produce most of the features of anaphylaxis presumably through their effect on vasoactive amine release, but much greater amounts of antibody are required as compared with the homocytotropic antibodies which mediate type I anaphylactic hypersensitivity. The increased vascular permeability which they generate helps the smaller complexes to become deposited in different parts of the vascular bed particularly in the capillaries of the kidney glomeruli where they may be seen to build up as 'lumpy' granules staining for antigen, immunoglobulin and complement (C3) by immunofluorescence (figure 6.9b) and as large amorphous masses associated with the

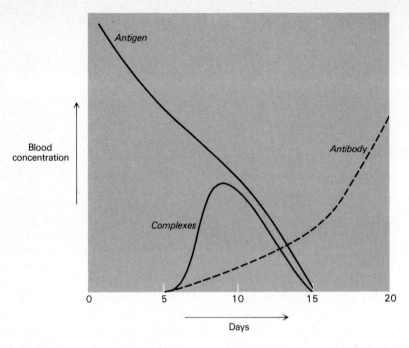

FIGURE 6.12. Formation of soluble complexes after injection of large amount of antigen (e.g. horse serum) as antibody is first synthesized. The complexes cause 'serum sickness'.

glomerular basement membrane in the electron microscope.

Experimentally, Dixon produced similar glomerular lesions by chronic administration of foreign proteins to rabbits. Not all animals showed the lesion and perhaps only those genetically capable of producing low affinity antibody (Soothill & Steward) or antibodies to a restricted number of determinants (Christian) formed soluble complexes. Preformed soluble complexes give rise to a transient glomerular lesion when injected into mice, but larger complexes tend to be taken up rapidly by the phagocytic cells before they can cause damage.

Many cases of glomerulonephritis are due to complexes and biopsies give a fluorescent staining pattern similar to that of figure 6.9b which depicts DNA/anti-DNA/complement deposits in the kidney of a patient with systemic lupus erythematosus (cf. chapter 9). Well known is the disease which can follow infection with certain strains of so-called 'nephritogenic' streptococci and the nephrotic syndrome of Nigerian children associated with malaria where complexes with antigens of the infecting organism have been implicated. Immune complex nephritis can arise in the course of chronic viral infections; for example, mice infected with lymphocytic choriomeningitis virus develop a glomerulonephritis associated with circulating complexes of virus and antibody. This may well represent a model for many cases of glomerulonephritis in man. The choroid plexus is also a favourite site for immune complex deposition and this could account for the frequency of central nervous disorders in systemic lupus. Neurologically affected patients tend to have depressed C4 in the cerebrospinal fluid and at post-mortem, SLE patients with neurological disturbances and high titre anti-DNA were shown to have scattered deposits of immunoglobulin and DNA in the choroid plexus. Subacute sclerosing panencephalitis is associated with a high c.s.f. to serum ratio of measles antibody and deposits containing Ig and measles Ag may be found in neural tissue.

The necrotizing arteritis produced in rabbits by experimental serum sickness closely resembles the histology of polyarteritis nodosa and it has recently been reported that in some of these patients, immune complexes containing the 'Australia antigen' (associated with hepatitis virus B) are present in the lesions. The extensive rashes of erythema nodosum associated with the lepromatous form of leprosy and perhaps with secondary syphilis probably have their root in the deposition of immune complexes involving antigens derived from these micro-organisms. Another example is the haemorrhagic shock syndrome found with some frequency in South-east Asia associated with Dengue virus infection. In some instances complexes formed with conjugates of body proteins with drugs such as penicillin give rise to hypersensitivity reactions.

If sera from patients with immune complex disease are kept at $4°$, many form a precipitate containing usually IgM and IgG. The IgM is an antiglobulin which is thought to bind to IgG itself perhaps acting as an antibody complexed with antigen. Indeed some authors have reported the presence of single strand DNA in cryoprecipitates obtained from patients with systemic lupus who are known to make DNA autoantibodies. Synovial fluids from rheumatoid arthritis patients commonly form immune cryoprecipitates of aggregated IgG with antiglobulin factors.

In general, immune complexes formed *in vivo* can be recognized by (i) immunofluorescent staining of tissue biopsies, (ii) their antigenic stimulation of antiglobulin and immuno-conglutin levels, and analysis of serum for (iii) abnormal peaks in the ultracentrifuge (iv) IgG in high molecular weight fractions on Sephadex gel filtration (v) precipitation with C1q or rheumatoid factors (vi) cryoprecipitation and (vii) inhibition

147

of K-cell activity *in vitro*. Because complement components are rapidly re-synthesized it is relatively unusual for serum levels to be significantly lowered; perhaps a more sensitive indicator of complement utilization by complexes is the appearance of C3 breakdown products immunoelectrophoretically identified as the β_{1A} and α_{2D} arcs (cf. figure 5.7).

Type IV—Cell-mediated (delayed-type) hypersensitivity

This form of hypersensitivity is encountered in many allergic reactions to bacteria, viruses and fungi, in the contact dermatitis resulting from sensitization to certain simple chemicals and in the rejection of transplanted tissues. Perhaps the best known example is the Mantoux reaction obtained by injection of tuberculin into the skin of an individual in whom previous infection with the mycobacterium had induced a state of cell-mediated immunity (CMI). The reaction is characterized by erythema and induration (figure 6.10c) which appears only after several hours (hence the term 'delayed') and reaches a maximum at 24–48 hours, thereafter subsiding. Histologically the earliest phase of the reaction is seen as a perivascular cuffing with mononuclear cells followed by a more extensive exudation of mono- and polymorphonuclear cells. The latter soon migrate out of the lesion leaving behind a predominantly mononuclear cell infiltrate consisting of lymphocytes and cells of the monocyte–macrophage series (figure 6.11b). This contrasts with the essentially 'polymorph' character of the Arthus reaction (figure 6.11a).

CELLULAR BASIS

Unlike the other forms of hypersensitivity which we have discussed, delayed-type reactivity cannot be transferred from a sensitive to a non-sensitized individual with serum antibody; lymphoid cells, in particular the small lymphocytes, are required. Thus a guinea-pig with negative skin reactions to tuberculin gives a positive response after injection of peritoneal exudate cells (containing lymphocytes and macrophages), lymph node cells, or peripheral blood cells from a donor previously sensitized to the tubercle bacillus (particularly if the donor and recipient are histocompatible so that the transferred cells are not rejected by a transplantation reaction). Transfer of delayed hypersensitivity has also been achieved in the human using viable blood white cells and interestingly, by a low molecular weight material extracted from them (Lawrence's transfer factor).

The defective cell-mediated hypersensitivity responses seen in children with thymic insufficiency and in thymectomized chickens, and the relatively unimpaired responses found in children with primary immunoglobulin deficiency and in bursectomized chickens clearly focuses attention on the thymus-dependent T-lymphocytes as the key cell population. In support of this view is the observation that sensitization of the skin with a chemical such as chlorodinitrobenzene which induces a predominantly delayed-type hypersensitivity state leads to an early proliferation and differentiation to blast forms of lymphocytes in the thymus dependent paracortical area of the lymph node. On the other hand, in mice injected with pneumococcus polysaccharide which stimulates antibody formation but not cell-mediated hypersensitivity, only the cortical lymphoid follicles show cellular changes, the paracortical areas remaining quiescent (cf. figure 3.6, p. 54).

The T-cells are antigen-sensitive (cf. chapter 3) and are thought to recognize their respective antigens by surface receptors, the nature of which is still hotly debated. Activated T-cells can bind exogenous immunoglobulin through the Fc region and the view is favoured that such immunoglobulin, probably in the form of a complex with antigen, is concerned in the mediation of T-cell co-operation and the formation of T-cell rosettes since both functions can be inhibited by anti-Ig sera. On the other hand, the balance of evidence has perhaps tended to swing against the idea that the T-cell bears an immunoglobulin receptor of *endogenous* origin on its surface, witness for example the failure to detect surface Ig on peripheral T-cells of completely bursectomized chickens using very sensitive techniques and the failure to inhibit T-cell cytotoxicity against allogeneic cells in culture by any anti-Ig serum so far available to immunologists. The fact that these cytotoxic cells show specificity for their target and can be adsorbed onto fibroblasts bearing the transplantation antigens to which the animal was originally sensitized (albeit by a mechanism unaffected by anti-Ig) clearly indicate that T-cells do have specific endogenous receptors even though we have as yet been unable to characterize them with any confidence.

The hypersensitivity reaction is probably initiated by antigen, which may be associated with or processed by a macrophage, combining with the receptors on the surface of appropriate T-lymphocytes present as memory cells following an earlier sensitization process. The cell membrane becomes activated and the signal is transmitted to the interior of the cell where the nucleus of the small lymphocyte with its compact chromatin appears to become derepressed; the cell transforms into a large blast cell and undergoes mitosis. At the same time a number of soluble factors are released which function as mediators of the ensuing hypersensitivity response.

EFFECTOR MECHANISMS

The supernatant fluid recovered after stimulating sensitized lymphocytes with antigen possesses several biological activities although the extent to which these may be ascribed to different molecular species is still unresolved. These factors have molecular weights of the order of 20,000–80,000 and are listed as follows.

(a) *Macrophage migration inhibition factor (MIF)*

The active migration of macrophages from a capillary tube is inhibited if MIF is present in the bathing tissue culture fluid. This is largely true whether or not antigen is present at this stage but evidence for an antigen-specific MIF has also been presented raising the admittedly speculative possibility that this might be specific T-cell receptor which is released on antigen stimulation and then binds to the surface of the macrophage. A somewhat analogous situation arises when T-cells interact with tumour cells to which they have been sensitized and release a factor (specific macrophage arming factor-SMAF; cf p. 194) which can endow macrophages with the power to selectively kill the tumour in question. Additionally the lymphokines produce significant morphological changes in the macrophages which become metabolically very active ('angry') and more effective in killing off ingested bacteria.

(b) *Monocyte chemotactic factor*

Monocytes will move across Millipore membranes towards higher concentrations of the factor.

(c) *Skin reactive factor*

This will initiate the exudation of cells when injected intra-dermally and may also increase capillary permeability.

(d) *Other biological activities*

Factors are also present which will evoke mitosis in uncommitted lymphocytes (?B-related to T-cell co-operation; cf p. 61) and which are cytotoxic, or at least growth inhibitory, for certain cultured cell lines. Preliminary evidence suggests the presence of a platelet aggregation factor and of interferon (? or a stimulator of interferon production by macrophages).

The amplifying effect of these factors probably accounts for the observation that after transfer of radiolabelled lymphoid cells from a sensitive donor to a normal recipient, only a very small percentage of the cells present in an antigen-induced skin hypersensitivity reaction are of donor origin. Evidently antigen activates a small number of the specifically sensitized donor cells randomly passing through the skin site and these are stimulated. The soluble factors gradually released as a result attract mononuclear cells, activate the macrophages and retain them in the lesion, and may also stimulate mitosis in uncommitted lymphocytes so giving rise to the typical histological appearance of a delayed-type reaction.

IN VITRO TESTS FOR CELL-MEDIATED
HYPERSENSITIVITY

Migration inhibition tests

The production of MIF by peritoneal exudate cells from sensitized guinea-pigs on incubation with antigen is widely accepted as an *in vitro* correlate of cell-mediated hypersensitivity. The cells are packed into capillary tubes which are placed in small tissue culture chambers. On incubation the macrophages migrate out to form a fan of cells on the bottom of the chamber. If specific antigen is present in the medium, MIF is produced and the migration is inhibited. The degree of inhibition is assessed from the area of the macrophage fan obtained in the presence of antigen expressed as a percentage of that in the control chambers lacking antigen (figure 6.13) and this correlates with the intensity of the delayed hypersensitivity state.

The macrophages act as non-specific indicators of the reaction between antigen and specifically sensitized lymphocytes. Thus a purified small lymphocyte population isolated from the peritoneal exudate of a sensitized pig is able to induce migration inhibition in the presence of antigen when mixed with as many as 50 times its number of macrophages taken from unsensitized

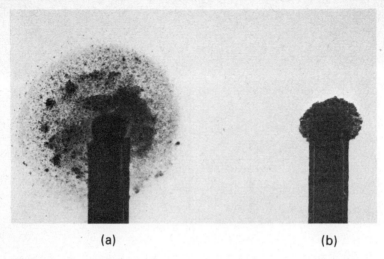

(a)   (b)

FIGURE 6.13. Migration inhibition as an *in vitro* test for cell-mediated hypersensitivity. Migration of peritoneal exudate cells from a sensitized guinea-pig: (a) control in absence of antigen and (b) in the presence of antigen. (Courtesy of Dr. J. Brostoff.)

animals; purified macrophages from the sensitized animal however are unable to produce MIF when mixed with lymphocytes from normal donors and incubated with antigen.

Greater difficulties have been encountered in attempting migration inhibition tests in the human. One variant is to incubate blood lymphocytes with antigen for several days and then to assay for MIF in the supernatant by addition to guinea-pig macrophages. Another is to mix the lymphocytes directly with the guinea-pig macrophages and to assess the effect of antigen on the migratory properties of the macrophages either in a MIF test or in the electric field of a cytopherometer. Inhibitory tests involving migration of buffy coat cells are potentially most useful but the conditions required to define when this represents a direct expression of T-cell reactivity have yet to be rigidly established.

Transformation

The proliferation of sensitized cells on contact with specific antigen and their change in morphology to larger blast-like cells with paler staining nuclei and basophilic cytoplasm (figure 3.5i, p. 53) has frequently been used as an *in vitro* test for cell-mediated hypersensitivity and several studies have shown reasonable correlation with *in vivo* results. The degree of stimulation is assessed either by the percentage of blast-like cells surviving in the culture or by the incorporation of labelled thymidine into newly synthesized DNA. The test is complicated by the possibility of recruitment into division of non-sensitized lymphocytes through release of a mitogenic factor from stimulated cells and also by the fact that B-lymphocytes may also be transformed.

Comparable changes can be induced in lymphocytes by certain plant mitogens of which the best known are phytohaemagglutinin (PHA) and concanavalin A (conA). These react with the cell surface non-specifically (i.e. not as an antigen) and produce the same series of cellular events as does antigen locking on to its specific surface receptor. Unlike the situation with antigen stimulation where only a small fraction of the cells are sensitive, PHA transforms the majority of the T-cells. Additionally a proportion of B-cells are affected although their response may prove to be T-cell dependent.

RELATION TO ANTIBODY SYNTHESIS

It was often thought that delayed sensitivity was a necessary stage in the process of humoral antibody synthesis. We now know that this is not really so. Pneumococcal polysaccharide in mice generates antibody synthesis but not CMI. Injection of certain antigens in soluble form followed by antigen in complete Freund's adjuvant selectively suppresses cellular rather than humoral immunity (immune deviation). Lastly, individuals lacking T-cells can still make antibodies, although not always so effectively. There is a link, however, in the co-operation of T- and B-cells (cf. chapter 3, p. 59) and if the same T-lymphocytes are capable of acting as effector cells for CMI and as co-operating cells for antibody production (figure 6.14), one might expect that factors which increase a state of CMI to a given antigen would correspondingly enhance antibody production in those instances where co-operation was a significant factor. Thus the finding of cell-mediated hypersensitivity in patients with atopic allergy may be a reflection of the fact that IgE antibodies to pollen and other allergens only tend to be formed in significant amounts when appropriately sensitized T-cells are available for co-operation. The increased antibody production to protein antigens incorporated in complete Freund's adjuvant (a water in oil emulsion containing killed tubercle bacilli) is partly due to an antigen depot effect, but may also be a consequence of the delayed-type hypersensitivity response evoked by this material since the specifically sensitized T-lymphocytes could enhance antibody synthesis

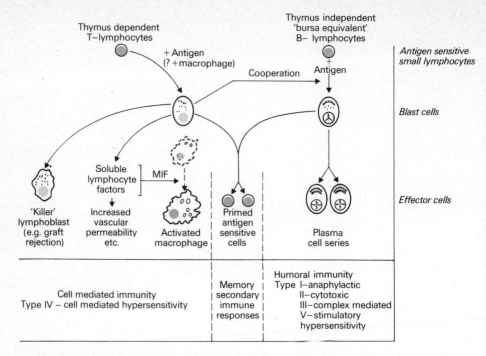

FIGURE 6.14. Relationship of B- and T-cell activity to different forms of hypersensitivity and immunity.

through co-operation. It may be recalled here that Freund's adjuvant is most effective in increasing the antibody response to antigens which are 'thymus dependent', i.e. where co-operation is required for a significant response.

TISSUE DAMAGE

Infection

The development of a state of cell-mediated hypersensitivity to bacterial products is probably responsible for the lesions associated with bacterial allergy such as the cavitation, caseation and general toxaemia seen in human tuberculosis and the granulomatous skin lesions found in patients with the tuberculoid form of leprosy. The skin rashes in smallpox and measles and the lesions of herpes simplex likewise have been attributed to a delayed-type allergic reaction to the virus. Cell-mediated hypersensitivity has also been demonstrated in the fungal diseases, dermatomycosis, coccidioidomycosis and histoplasmosis, and in the protozoal diseases, leishmaniasis and schistosomiasis. The relationship to cell-mediated *immunity* is discussed in the following chapter.

154

Contact dermatitis

The dermal route of inoculation tends to favour the development of a T-cell response and delayed-type reactions are often produced by foreign materials capable of binding to body constituents to form new antigens. Thus contact hypersensitivity can occur in people who become sensitized while working with chemicals such as picryl chloride and chromates, or who repeatedly come into contact with the substance urushiol from the poison ivy plant. *p*-Phenylene diamine in certain hair dyes, neomycin in topically applied ointments and nickel salts formed from articles such as nickel suspenders can provoke similar reactions.

Other examples

Delayed hypersensitivity contributes significantly to the prolonged reactions which result from insect bites. Another example is provided by the cytotoxic effects of activated T-lymphocytes on their target cells in a homograft undergoing rejection and this is discussed in chapter 8 together with its possible implication for the control of cancer cells. The contribution made by cell-mediated hypersensitivity reactions to different autoimmune diseases is even now rather uncertain (chapter 9).

Type V—Stimulatory hypersensitivity

Many cells receive instruction by agents such as hormones through surface receptors which specifically bind the external agent presumably through complementarity of structure. This combination may lead to allosteric changes in configuration of the receptor or of adjacent molecules which become activated and transmit a signal to the cell interior. For example, when thyroid stimulating hormone (TSH) of pituitary origin binds to the thyroid cell receptors there appears to be an activation of adenyl cyclase in the membrane which generates cyclic-AMP from ATP and this substance acts to stimulate activity in the thyroid cell. The long acting thyroid stimulator (LATS; chapter 9) is an autoantibody probably directed against an antigen on the thyroid surface which stimulates the cell and produces the same changes as TSH, similarly utilizing the cyclic-AMP pathway. It is likely that the LATS antibody combines with a site on the TSH receptor or an adjacent molecule

Summary of different types of hypersensitivity

TABLE 6.1. Comparison of different types of hypersensitivity

	I Anaphylactic	II Cytotoxic	III Complex-mediated	IV Cell-mediated	V Stimulatory
Antibody mediating reaction	Homocytotropic Ab Mast-cell binding	Humoral Ab ±CF*	Humoral Ab ±CF	'Ab' bound to T-lymphocyte	Humoral Ab Non-CF
Antigen	Usually exogenous (e.g. grass pollen)	Cell surface	Extracellular	Extracellular or cell surface	Cell surface
Response to intradermal antigen:					
Max. reaction	30 min.	—	3–8 hr.	24–48 hr.	—
Appearance	Wheal and flare	—	Erythema and oedema	Erythema and induration	—
Histology	Degranulated mast cells; oedema; eosinophils	—	Acute inflammatory reaction; predominant polymorphs	Perivascular inflammation: polymorphs migrate out leaving predominantly mononuclear cells	—
Transfer sensitivity to normal subject	←————— Serum antibody —————→			Lymphoid cells Transfer factor	Serum antibody
Examples:	Atopic allergy, e.g. hay fever	Haemolytic disease of newborn (Rh)	Complex glomerulonephritis Farmer's lung	Mantoux reaction to TB Skin homograft rejection	Thyrotoxicosis (LATS)

* CF = Complement fixation.

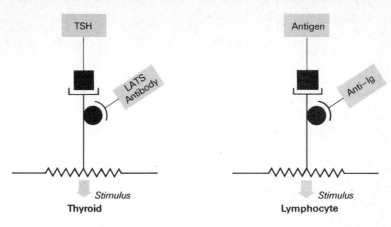

FIGURE 6.15. Stimulation of thyroid cell and of lymphocyte by physiological agent or by antibody both of which cause comparable membrane changes leading to cell activation.

to produce the allosteric change required for adenyl cyclase activation. The situation is analogous to lymphocyte stimulation; the small lymphocytes with immunoglobulin surface receptors can be stimulated by changes induced through the receptor molecules either by binding of specific antigen or by an antibody to the immunoglobulin (even anti-Fc) as shown in figure 6.15. Other experimental examples of stimulation by antibodies to cell surface antigens may be cited: the transformation of lymphocytes by heterologous anti-lymphocyte serum (ALS); the induction of pinocytosis by anti-macrophage serum; and the mitogenic effect of antibodies to sea-urchin eggs. It is worthy of note that although antibodies to enzymes directed against determinants near to the active site can exert a blocking effect, combination with more distant determinants can sometimes bring about allosteric conformational changes which are associated with a considerable increase in enzymic activity as has been described for certain variants of penicillinase and β-galactosidase.

Further reading

Bloom B.R. & Glade P.R. (eds.) (1971) *In vitro Methods in Cell Mediated Immunity*. Acad. Press.
Brondz B.D. (1972) Lymphocyte receptors and mechanisms of in vitro cell-mediated immune reactions. *Transplant.Rev.*, **10**, 112.
Brostoff J. (1973) Atopic allergy. *Brit.J.Hosp.Med.*, **9**, p. 29.
Cochrane C.G. & Koffler D. (1973) Immune complex disease in experimental animals and man. *Adv.in Immunology*, **16**, 186.

Gell P.G.H., Coombs R.A. & Lachmann P. (eds.) (1974) *Clinical Aspects of Immunology*, 3rd ed., Section IV. Blackwell Scientific Publications, Oxford.

Ling N.R. (1968) *Lymphocyte Stimulation*. North Holland, Amsterdam.

Mollison P.L. (1970) Red cell destruction. *Brit.J.Haematol.*, **18**, 249.

Pepys J. (1969) *Hypersensitivity Diseases of the Lungs due to Fungi and Organic Dusts*. Karger, Basle.

Perlmann P., Perlmann H. & Wigzell H. (1972) Lymphocyte medicated cytotoxicity in vitro. Induction and inhibition by humoral antibody and nature of effector cells. *Transpl.Rev.*, **13**, 91.

Stanworth D.S. (1973) *Immediate Hypersensitivity*. North Holland, Amsterdam.

Turk J.L. (1967) *Delayed Hypersensitivity*. North Holland, Amsterdam.

Turk J.L. (1973) *Immunology in Clinical Medicine*. Heinemann, London.

(1967) Delayed hypersensitivity: specific cell-mediated immunity. *Brit.med. Bull.*, **23**, No. 1.

(1971) Symposium on Immune Complexes and Diseases. *J.Exp.Med.*, **134**, Supplement.

7 Immunity to infection

Our resistance to infection by the myriad micro-organisms which surround us is based upon 'non-specific' factors which can act independently of the immune system, and specifically acquired immunity (table 7.1) which frequently operates in concert with these 'non-specific' factors, thereby greatly increasing their effectiveness.

Non-specific immunity

Aside from ill-understood constitutional factors which make one species innately susceptible and another resistant to certain infections, a number of 'non-specific' antimicrobial mechanisms have been recognized. For example, most bacteria fail to survive for long on the skin because of the direct inhibitory effects of lactic acid and fatty acids in sweat and sebaceous secretions and the low pH which they generate. Ciliated epithelium in the respiratory tree acts to prevent the bulk of the inhaled dust particles with their associated organisms from reaching the alveoli. Mucus secretions can inhibit the penetration of cells by viruses through competition with cell surface receptors for the viral neuraminidase. The bactericidal enzyme

TABLE 7.1. Mechanisms of resistance to infection

Type	Examples
Non-specific immunity	Phagocytosis—lysozyme—interferon
Specifically acquired immunity	
Passive — Natural	Maternally derived Ig in baby
Passive — Induced	Protection by preformed heterologous antibody or homologous γ-globulin
Active — Natural	Exposure to infection
Active — Induced	Immunization with toxoid, or killed or attenuated organisms

lysozyme is abundantly present in such secretions (e.g. tears and saliva) and in the granules of polymorphs and macrophages, and is widely distributed throughout the body fluids.

Bacteria can be removed by *phagocytosis*. They adhere to polymorphs and macrophages by some rather primitive recognition mechanism on the part of the phagocytic cells; the microbes are then engulfed into a phagosome by arms of cytoplasm which wrap around them. The phagosome then fuses with a lysosomal granule to form a phagolysosome in which the bacterium is slaughtered by a battery of factors: low pH, a whole variety of hydrolytic enzymes including lysozyme and a number of bactericidal basic polypeptides (figure 7.1). The importance of polymorph kill is emphasized by the seriousness of chronic granulomatous disease and the Chediak–Higashi syndrome in children who have defective neutrophil leucocytes which ingest but cannot kill bacteria and who are as a result susceptible to chronic infections.

The acute inflammatory response to foreign organisms and to the products of any tissue injury caused by them also has a beneficial protective role. The increased capillary permeability leads to the egress of polymorphs and later of monocytes from the blood stream into the site where they combat the microbes by phagocytosis, and to the massive transudation of serum bactericidal factors. These include:

(a) *C-reactive protein*, a molecule unrelated to the immunoglobulins which precipitates with the group-specific C-carbohydrate of pneumococci in the presence of Ca^{2+}, and

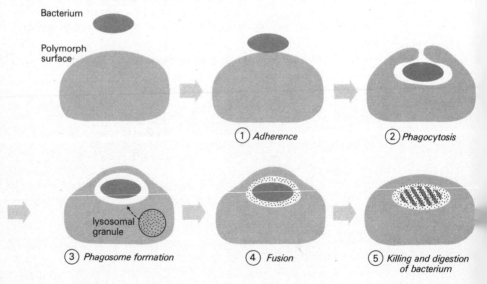

FIGURE 7.1. Phagocytosis of bacterium by neutrophil leucocyte.

(b) *properdin* and the *complement system* which together can kill a variety of micro-organisms in the presence of Mg^{2+} through activation of the alternative pathway (p. 122).

The so-called '*natural antibodies*' present in the serum of normal individuals are largely IgM and almost certainly appear as a response to repeated contact with the many bacterial antigens presented by the gut flora. As might be expected they are only present in very low titre in animals reared under germ-free conditions. In any event they should more correctly be considered under the heading of specifically acquired immunity.

Lastly we should include the non-specific antiviral agent *interferon* which inhibits intracellular viral replication and is itself synthesized by cells in response to viral infection. Viral interference, the resistance of an animal or cell infected with one virus to superinfection with a second unrelated virus, may be attributed to interferon. In children given live measles vaccine, smallpox vaccine will not take if inoculated at the height of interferon production. It must be presumed that interferon plays a significant role in the recovery from, as distinct from the prevention of viral infections; however the difficulties encountered by children with T-cell deficiencies (see below under 'Immunodeficiency Disorders') in coping with viral infections indicates that if interferon is the major factor in recovery it must be connected in some way with the operation of cell-mediated immune mechanisms.

This raises a more general point: the non-specific defence mechanisms are of vital importance but the experience with children lacking either B- or T-lymphocyte systems is clear proof that the development of specific acquired immune responsiveness is indispensable for survival in normal individuals. We shall now consider the ways in which protection against infection is conferred by these specific immunological responses and the manner in which they operate to augment the non-specific mechanisms.

Immunity to bacterial infection

ROLE OF HUMORAL ANTIBODY

Phagocytosis

Adherence of bacteria to phagocytic cells is necessary before the organisms can be engulfed and digested. Many virulent microbes such as the encapsulated forms of pneumococci do not stick readily to these cells but are rapidly phagocytosed when coated with specific antibody as may be seen by following the rate of disappearance of coated and uncoated bacteria from the blood stream (figure 7.2). The rate of disappearance of coated organisms is somewhat reduced in animals depleted of complement (figure 7.2). The role of antibody and complement in 'opsonizing' bacteria (cf. pp. 116 & 122) is mediated through specific receptors on the phagocytic cell surface which have a high affinity for IgG (particularly subclasses 1 and 3 in the human) and for the C3b component of complement (figure 7.3).

Bacteria may also be captured by antibody already fixed to the macrophage receptor site (cytophilic antibody). However, it is probable that adherence is mediated more through opsonization than through the prior binding of cytophilic antibody to the macrophage (figure 7.4).

Adherence to polymorphs and to the fixed cells of the reticulo-endothelial system probably involves comparable mechanisms.

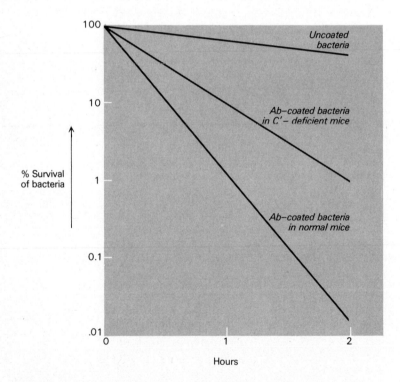

FIGURE 7.2. Effect of opsonizing antibody and complement on rate of clearance of virulent bacteria from the blood. The uncoated bacteria are not readily phagocytosized but on coating with antibody, adherence to phagocytes is increased many-fold. The adherence is somewhat less effective in animals temporarily depleted of complement.

162

Complexes containing C3 may also show immune adherence to primate red cells and rabbit platelets to provide phagocytosable aggregates.

Some strains of Gram-negative bacteria which have a lipoprotein outer wall resembling mammalian surface membranes in structure are susceptible to the bactericidal action of fresh serum containing antibody. The antibody initiates the development of a complement mediated lesion producing similar 'holes' to those caused by complement in mammalian cells (cf. figure 5.23); this allows access of serum lysozyme to the inner wall of the bacterium with resulting cell death. Activation of complement through union of antibody and bacterium will also generate the C3a and C5a anaphylatoxins leading to extensive transudation of serum components including more antibody, and to the chemotactic attraction of polymorphs to aid in phagocytosis.

The mechanisms by which IgA antibodies afford protection in the external body fluids, tears, saliva, nasal secretions and those bathing the surfaces of the intestine (so-called 'copro-antibodies') and lung is not yet fully elucidated; synergistic action with lysozyme and complement has been reported in some instances and it remains a possibility that the secretory

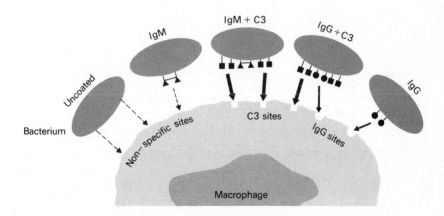

FIGURE 7.3. Immunoglobulin and complement coats greatly increase the adherence of bacteria (and other antigens) to macrophages and polymorphs. Uncoated or IgM (⊢▲⊣) coated bacteria adhere relatively weakly to non-specific sites but there are specific receptors for IgG (Fc) (●) and C3 (▲) on the macrophage surface which considerably enhance the strength of binding. The augmenting effect of complement is due to the fact that two adjacent IgG molecules can fix many C3 molecules (cf. 'bonus' effect of multivalency; p. 15). Although IgM does not bind specifically to the macrophage, it promotes adherence through complement fixation.

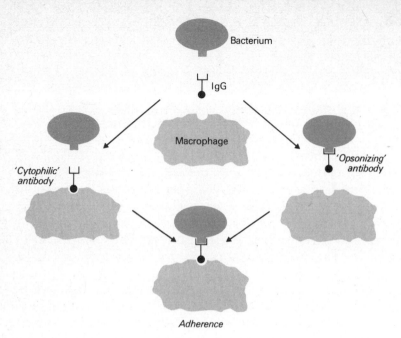

Bacterium

IgG

Macrophage

'Cytophilic'
antibody

'Opsonizing'
antibody

Adherence

FIGURE 7.4. Cytophilic and opsonizing antibody provide alternative
mechanisms for promoting adherence of bacteria to macrophages. A
bacterium in serum will select its specific antibody and become coated with
it thereby offering a highly multivalent moiety for opsonic binding to the
phagocyte. In contrast, the specific antibody present on the phagocyte as a
cytophilic Ig is heavily diluted by other antibodies of irrelevant specificity
and the multivalency of the link to the bacterium will be substantially
lower. On these grounds one would predict the opsonizing route to be the
most significant.

component of the IgA dimers will prove to have some biological
activity. It appears that the adherence of bacteria to mucosal
surfaces is inhibited by specific IgA antibody and this would
certainly help to deny the organisms access to the body tissues.

Neutralization of toxins

In addition to their role in removal of microbes, antibodies act
to neutralize the soluble exotoxins (e.g. phospholipase C of
Clostridium welchii) released by bacteria. Combination near the
biologically active site of the toxin would stereochemically
block reaction with the substrate, particularly if it were macro-
molecular; combination distant from the active site may also
cause inhibition through allosteric conformational changes. In
its complex with antibody, the toxin may be unable to diffuse
away rapidly and will be susceptible to phagocytosis, especially
if the complex can be increased in size by the action of naturally

occurring antibodies to altered IgG (antiglobulin factors) and altered C3 (immunoconglutinin).

ROLE OF CELL-MEDIATED IMMUNITY (CMI)

Some strains of bacteria such as the tubercle and leprosy bacilli, and listeria and brucella organisms, are able to live and continue their growth within the cytoplasm of macrophages after their uptake by phagocytosis. In an elegant series of experiments, Mackaness has demonstrated the importance of CMI reactions for the killing of these intracellular facultative parasites and the establishment of an immune state. Animals infected with moderate doses of *M. tuberculosis* overcome the infection and are immune to subsequent challenge with the bacillus. Surprisingly, if they are given an unrelated organism such as *Listeria monocytogenes* at *the same time* as the second infection with tubercle bacillus, they are resistant and can kill the listeria which have been engulfed by macrophages. Without the prior immunity to *M. tuberculosis* or the second challenge with this organism, the animal would have succumbed to listeria infection. In the same way, an animal immune to listeria can rapidly kill tubercle bacilli given at the same time as a second infection with listeria (table 7.2). Thus the triggering of a specific secondary immune response to one organism may endow the animal with a simultaneous but transient non-specific resistance to unrelated microbes of similar growth habits.

Immunity—both specific and non-specific—can be transferred to a normal recipient with lymphocytes but not macrophages or serum from an immune animal (figure 7.5). This strongly suggests that the specific immunity is mediated by T-cells. In support of this view is the greater susceptibility to

TABLE 7.2. Induction of non-specific immunity by a CMI reaction

Primary Infection:	Tubercle bacillus			Nothing	Listeria
Challenge:	Tubercle bacillus	Listeria	Tubercle bacillus + Listeria	Tubercle bacillus + Listeria	Tubercle bacillus + Listeria
Result:	**Immune**	Infection	**Immune**	Infection	**Immune**

infection with tubercle and leprosy bacilli of mice in which the T-lymphocytes have been depressed by thymectomy plus anti-lymphocyte serum (see chapter 8). In human leprosy, the disease presents as a spectrum ranging from the *tuberculoid* form with very few viable organisms, to the *lepromatous* form characterized by an abundance of *Mycobacterium leprae* within the macrophages. As Turk has emphasized, the tuberculoid state is associated with an active T-lymphocyte system giving good PHA transformation of lymphocytes and cell-mediated dermal hypersensitivity responses. In the lepromatous form, there is poor T-cell reactivity and the paracortical areas in the lymph nodes are depleted of lymphocytes although there are numerous plasma cells which contribute to a high level of circulating antibody. Clearly CMI rather than humoral immunity is important for the control of the leprosy bacillus.

The non-specific immunity to intracellular facultative bacteria described above can be induced by any cell-mediated

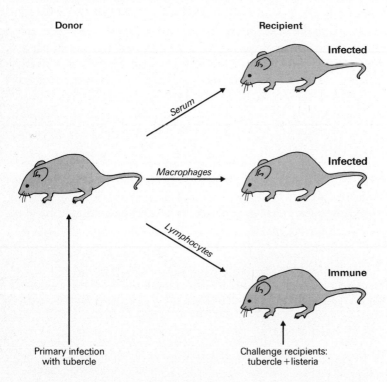

FIGURE 7.5. Transfer of specific and non-specific immunity by lymphocytes from an immune animal. The syngeneic recipient of the lymphocytes resisted simultaneous challenge with tubercle and listeria organisms. The recipients were not immune to listeria given without the tubercle. Serum or macrophages were ineffective in transferring immunity (after Mackaness).

hypersensitivity reaction. For example, guinea-pigs previously sensitized with bovine γ-globulin (BGG) in complete Freund's adjuvant, are resistant to challenge with brucella given at the same time as BGG. Animals also show non-specific immunity to such organisms during a graft vs. host reaction (see chapter 8).

Macrophages in different states of development probably vary in their ability to kill these microbes after ingestion. Perhaps the less mature cells with few hydrolytic granules are susceptible and support the growth of intracellular bacteria. It seems likely that during a CMI reaction when sensitized T-lymphocytes are stimulated by contact with specific antigen, one of the many soluble factors released (? MIF—chapter 6) may confer on these macrophages the power to kill the ingested organisms. Thus the specificity lies at the level of the initial reaction of T-cell with its antigen; the non-specific immunity arises from the newly acquired ability of the macrophage to kill *any* organism it has phagocytosed (figure 7.6). Macrophages taken from animals with graft vs. host reactions where the grafted T-lymphocytes react against the host appear to be very active when examined *in vitro*; these 'angry' macrophages have very motile cytoplasmic processes and show well-developed intracellular granules. Similar changes have been induced in

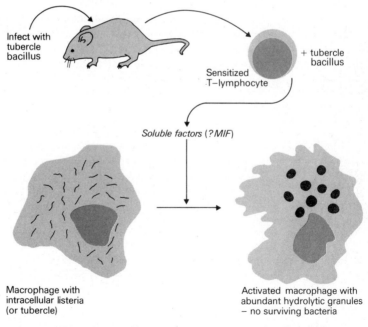

FIGURE 7.6. Macrophage killing of intracellular bacteria triggered by specific cell-mediated immunity reaction. (The final stage shown is probable but still hypothetical.)

ordinary macrophage cultures treated with supernatants containing MIF obtained by incubating sensitized T-cells with antigen, and it would be expected that the treated macrophages would be able to digest phagocytosed listeria and similar organisms.

Immunity to viral infection

Serum antibody

Antibody can neutralize viruses by stereochemically inhibiting their combination with the receptor site on cells to prevent infection and subsequent multiplication, and by enhancing their phagocytosis and intracellular digestion through the mechanisms already described under humoral immunity to bacteria. Relatively low concentrations of circulating antibody can be effective and one is familiar with the protection afforded by poliomyelitis antibodies, and by human γ-globulin given prophylactically to individuals exposed to measles. The most clear-cut protection is seen in diseases with long incubation times where the virus has to travel through the blood stream before it reaches the tissue which it finally infects. For example, in poliomyelitis the virus gains access to the body via the gastrointestinal tract and eventually passes through the circulation to reach the brain cells which become infected. The prolonged period before the virus infects the brain allows time for a secondary immune response in a primed host which effectively protects against disease.

Local factors

With other viral diseases, such as influenza and the common cold, there is a short incubation time related to the fact that the final target organ for the virus is the same as the portal of entry and no intermediate stage involving passage through the body occurs. There is little time for a primary antibody response to be mounted and in all likelihood the rapid production of interferon is the most significant mechanism used to counter the viral infection. Experimental studies certainly indicate that after an early peak of interferon production, there is a rapid fall in the titre of live virus in the lungs of mice infected with influenza (figure 7.7). Antibody, as assessed by the *serum* titre, seems to arrive on the scene much too late to be of value in aiding recovery. However, recent investigations have shown that antibody levels may be elevated in the *local* fluids bathing the infected surfaces, e.g. nasal mucosa and lung, despite low serum titres and it is the production of antiviral antibody (most prominently IgA) by locally deployed immunologically primed cells which may prove to be of great importance for the *prevention* of subsequent infection. Unfortunately, in so far as the common cold is concerned, a subsequent infection is likely to involve an antigenically unrelated virus so that general immunity to colds is difficult to achieve.

Cell-mediated immunity

Yet another factor must be considered. Children with primary immunodeficiency (see below) affecting the operation of the T-lymphocyte system have difficulty in coping with certain viral infections such as smallpox, whereas patients with immunoglobulin deficiency and intact cell-mediated immunity mechanisms are not troubled in this way. It is still not exactly clear how CMI contributes to recovery from viral infection but a collaborative role with macrophages mediated by antigen-induced T-cell lymphokines must be involved (cf. p. 130). The chemotactic factor attracts mononuclear phagocytes to the site

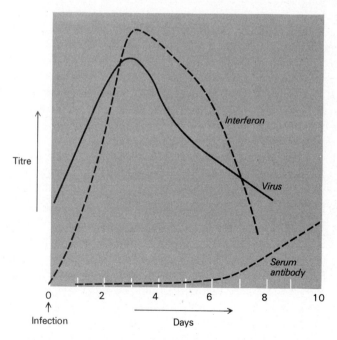

FIGURE 7.7. Appearance of interferon and serum Ab in relation to recovery from influenze virus infection of the lungs of mice (from Isaacs A., *New Scientist* 1961, **11**, 81).

of T-cell interaction with antigen where they become activated and also stimulated to produce interferon. Macrophages are known to phagocytize and kill certain viruses (e.g. mouse pox) and somehow prevent their spread from cell to cell. Furthermore, the viruses susceptible to CMI—pox, herpes and leukaemogenic viruses—give rise to new antigens on the surface of infected cells and one would expect these cells to be destroyed by sensitized T-cells as though they were foreign grafts. Lastly we should not overlook the helper effect of the T-cells for antibody production which also fulfils a protective role in the ways discussed above.

Immunity to parasitic infections

PROTOZOA

After recovery from parasitic infection, the organisms may be completely eradicated and the host remains solidly immune to reinfection: we speak of a *sterile immunity*. Often the parasites are not completely eliminated but small numbers continue to be harboured even though the host is able to resist superinfection; this state is referred to by parasitologists as *premunition*. The precise immunological mechanisms which operate in premunition are still not completely understood. Neither have the relative roles of humoral antibody or cell-mediated immunity been clearly established in relation to the defence against protozoal parasites. Perhaps the generalization may be made that a humoral response develops when the organisms invade the blood-stream (malaria, trypanosomiasis) whereas CMI is usually elicited by parasites which develop in the tissues (e.g. cutaneous leishmaniasis).

Circulating antibodies have often been shown to offer protection against the blood-borne forms but the parasites can be wily. Thus in toxoplasmosis, although antibody is protective it cannot eliminate the cystic stage; as a result the overt clinical disease is rare but subclinical infection is relatively frequent. In trypanosomiasis and malaria, the parasites escape from the cytocidal action of humoral antibody on their cycling blood forms by the ingenious trick of altering their antigenic constitution. Figure 7.8 illustrates how the trypanosome continues to infect the host, even after fully protective antibodies appear, by *antigenic variation* to a form which these antibodies cannot inactivate; as antibodies to the new antigens are synthesized, the parasite escapes again by changing to yet a further variant and so on. This may explain why in hyperendemic areas,

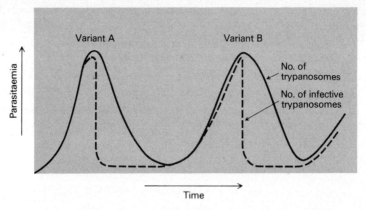

FIGURE 7.8. Antigenic variation during chronic trypanosome infection.
As antibody to the initial variant A is formed, the blood trypanosomes
become complexed prior to phagocytosis and are no longer infective leaving
a small number of viable parasites which have acquired a new antigenic
constitution. This new variant (B) now multiplies until it, too, is
neutralized by the primary antibody response and is succeeded by variant
C (after Gray A.R., see further reading list).

children are subjected to repeated attacks of malaria for their
first few years and are then solidly immune to further infection.
Immunity must presumably be developed against all the antigenic variants before full protection can be attained, and indeed
it is known that IgG from individuals with solid immunity can
effectively terminate malaria infections in young children.

Cell-mediated immunity is directly concerned in the recovery from certain
forms of leishmaniasis but studies on laboratory models have not so far
defined all the factors involved. For example, cultured guinea pig macrophages activated by the Mackaness phenomenon so that they non-specifically
kill ingested listeria (cf. p. 165), take up *Leishmania enrietti* and allow the
organisms to grow. Similarly, activated mouse macrophages which have
ingested *Toxoplasma gondii* allow growth through a failure to effect lysosome
fusion with the phagosome containing the organism. Almost certainly a
further antigen-specific factor, either cytophilic antibody or perhaps specific
macrophage arming factor (p. 150) is required to help the macrophage deal
with the parasite; in other words the simple idea that a non-specifically
activated macrophage will always kill *any* organism growing within its cytoplasm is going to need some amendment.

HELMINTHS

A marked feature of the immune reaction to helminthic infections such as *Trichinella spiralis* in man and *Nippostrongylus
brasiliensis* in the rat is the high level of homocytotropic (reaginic) antibody produced. In man serum levels of IgE can rise

from normal values of around 100 ng/ml to as high as 10,000 ng/ml. This exceptional increase has encouraged the view that IgE represents an important line of defence. One suggestion is that histamine released by contact of antigen with IgE-coated mast cells can aid the expulsion of the worm from the gut. Another view is that such a local anaphylactic reaction in the gut may lead to exudation of serum proteins known to contain high concentrations of protective antibodies in all the major immunoglobulin classes.

Schistosomiasis presents another intriguing situation. The adult worm lives permanently within the mesenteric vessels of the host, despite the fact that the blood which bathes it contains antibodies which can prevent a second infection. Smithers and Terrey have shown that the parasites make themselves resistant to these immune processes by disguising themselves with an outer coat of the host's antigens!

Summary of interactions between non-specific and adaptive immunity

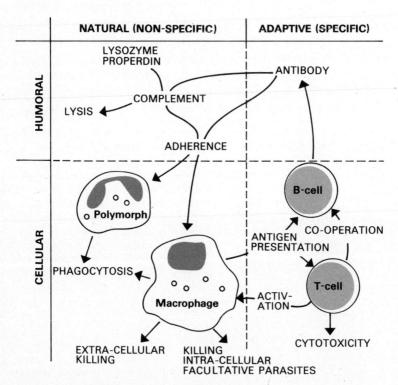

FIGURE 7.9. Simplified scheme to emphasize the interactions between natural and specific immunity mechanisms (based on Playfair J.H.L. (1974) *Brit.Med.Bull.*, **30**, 24).

Prophylaxis

PASSIVELY ACQUIRED IMMUNITY

Temporary protection against infection can be established by giving preformed antibody from another individual of the same or a different species. As the acquired antibodies are utilized by combination with antigen or catabolized in the normal way, this protection is gradually lost.

Homologous antibodies

Maternal. In the first few months of life while the baby's own lymphoid system is slowly getting under way, protection is afforded by maternally derived antibodies acquired by placental transfer and by intestinal absorption of colostral immuno-globulins.

γ-Globulin. Preparations of pooled human adult γ-globulin are of value to modify the effects of measles, particularly in individuals with defective immune responses such as premature infants, children with primary immunodeficiency or patients on steroid treatment. Contacts with cases of infectious hepatitis and smallpox may also be afforded protection by γ-globulin, especially when in the latter case the material is derived from the serum of individuals vaccinated some weeks previously. Human anti-tetanus immunoglobulin is preferable to horse antitoxin which can cause serum reactions.

Isolated γ-globulin preparations tend to form small aggregates spontaneously and these can lead to severe anaphylactic reactions when administered intravenously on account of their ability to aggregate platelets and to activate complement and generate C3a and C5a anaphylatoxins. For this reason the material is always injected intramuscularly. Preparations free of aggregates would be welcome as would separate pools with raised antibody titres to selected organisms such as vaccinia, *Herpes zoster*, tetanus and perhaps rubella.

Heterologous antibodies

Horse globulins containing anti-tetanus and anti-diphtheria toxins have been extensively employed prophylactically, but at the present time the practice is more restricted because of the complication of serum sickness developing in response to the foreign protein. This is more likely to occur in subjects already sensitized by previous contact with horse globulin; thus individuals who have been given horse anti-tetanus (e.g. for immediate protection after receiving a wound out in the open) are later advised to undergo a course of active immunization to obviate the need for further injections of horse protein in any subsequent emergency.

ACTIVE IMMUNIZATION

The objective of vaccination is to provide effective immunity by establishing adequate levels of antibody and a primed population of cells which can rapidly expand on renewed contact with antigen. The first contact with antigen during vaccination obviously should not be injurious and the manoeuvre is to modify the pathogenic effect without losing important antigens:

(a) *Toxoids*. Bacterial exotoxins such as those produced by diphtheria and tetanus bacilli can be successfully detoxified by formaldehyde treatment without destroying the major immunogenic determinants (figure 7.10). Immunization with the *toxoid* will therefore provoke the formation of protective antibodies. The toxoid is generally given after adsorption to aluminium hydroxide which acts as an adjuvant, perhaps by efficient presentation of antigen to the macrophage system, and produces higher antibody titres.

(b) *Killed organisms*. Dead bacteria and viruses which have been inactivated provide a safe antigen for immunization. Examples are typhoid, which may be combined with relatively ineffective paratyphoid A and B, cholera and killed poliomyelitis (Salk) vaccines. The immunity conferred by killed vaccines is often inferior to that resulting from infection with live organisms. This must be partly because the replication of the living microbes confronts the host with a larger and more

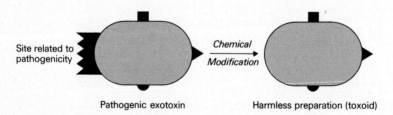

Site related to pathogenicity

Chemical Modification

Pathogenic exotoxin

Harmless preparation (toxoid)

FIGURE 7.10. Modification of toxin to harmless toxoid without losing many of the antigenic determinants (■ ● ▲). Thus antibodies to the toxoid will react well with the original toxin. Utilizing a similar principle, micro-organisms can be rendered harmless by killing or attenuating to non-virulent but still living forms.

sustained dose of antigen and also because the immune response takes place largely at the site of the natural infection. As an example cholera infection will be most efficiently dealt with by antibodies produced locally by the gut wall ('copro-antibodies') yet injected *killed* vaccine may stimulate antibody synthesis in the spleen and perhaps many lymph nodes without initiating an adequate response in the intestinal lymphoid system. Ideally immunity would be best established by infection with a modified but live (attenuated) form of cholera bacillus which would multiply at the site of the natural infection without producing disease. Prolongation of antigen exposure with dead vaccines has been attempted using water in oil emulsions (cf. incomplete Freund's adjuvant) but their use is not encouraged because of occasional formation of nodules and sterile abscesses at the injection site and also the knowledge that incomplete Freund's adjuvant is an excellent agent for inducing tumours in mice.

(c) *Attenuated organisms*. We have discussed the advantages of vaccinating with live non-virulent forms. Pasteur first achieved attenuation of chicken cholera bacillus and anthrax by such artifices as culture at higher temperatures and under anaerobic conditions, and was able to confer immunity by infection with the attenuated organisms. A virulent strain of *Mycobacterium tuberculosis* became attenuated by chance in 1908 when Calmette and Guérin at the Institut Pasteur, Lille, added bile to the culture medium in an attempt to achieve dispersed growth. After 13 years of culture in bile-containing medium, the strain remained attenuated and was used successfully to vaccinate children against tuberculosis. The same organism, BCG (Bacille, Calmette, Guérin), is widely used today for immunization of tuberculin negative individuals; it may also bestow a reasonable degree of protection against *Mycobacterium leprae*.

Attenuated vaccines for poliomyelitis (Sabin), measles and rubella have gained general acceptance. The possibility of reversion to a virulent form is always present with the use of attenuated organisms; to some extent this eventuality can be countered by use of immunoglobulin preparations containing reasonable titres of the appropriate antibodies.

Some general problems

Vigorous public health immunization programmes have virtually eliminated diseases like diphtheria, smallpox and poliomyelitis from many communities. With certain vaccines there is a very small, but still real, risk of developing complications such as encephalitis and this must be balanced against the expected risk of contracting the disease. Where this is slight, some may prefer to avoid general vaccination and to rely upon a crash course backed up if necessary by passive immunization in the localities around isolated outbreaks of infectious disease.

It is important to recognize those children with immuno-deficiency before injection of live organisms; a child with impaired T-cell reactivity can become overwhelmed by BCG and die. The extent to which children with partial deficiencies are at risk has yet to be assessed.

A worrying feature of immunization with viruses grown on monkey kidney culture is the presence of simian viruses which could be potentially oncogenic; SV-40, for example, is known to cause transformation of human cells in culture. More attention is being paid to the use of human diploid cell lines as viral hosts in the hope that this will limit the risk of oncogenic virus contamination.

One should mention the difficulty in producing adequate vaccines for respiratory viruses because of the multitude of antigenic variants which arise. Problems stemming from the competition of several antigens used concurrently in multiple vaccines, and the possible deviating influence of maternally derived antibody have been discussed in earlier chapters.

The current schedule of vaccination and immunization procedures followed in this country are given in the Appendix.

Primary immunodeficiency

The most clear-cut, and correspondingly rare, examples of extreme immunodeficiency in children are documented in table 7.3.

TABLE 7.3. Extreme examples of primary immunodeficiency in children

Deficiency	Example	Immune Response		Infection	Treatment
		Humoral	Cellular		
B-cell	Infantile sex-linked a-γ-globulinaemia (Bruton)	↓↓	Normal	Pyogenic bacteria Pneumocystis carinii Candida	γ-Globulin
T-cell	Thymic hypoplasia (DiGeorge)	↓	↓↓	Certain viruses Candida	Thymus graft
Stem cell	Severe combined deficiency (Swiss-type)	↓↓	↓↓	All the above	Bone marrow graft

1. B-cell deficiency

The production of immunoglobulin is grossly depressed and there are few lymphoid follicles or plasma cells in lymph node biopsies. The children are subject to repeated infection by pyogenic ('pus-forming') bacteria—*Staphylococcus aureus, Streptococcus pyogenes and pneumoniae, Neisseria meningitidis, Haemophilus influenzae*—and by *Candida albicans* (thrush) and a rare protozoon, *Pneumocystis carinii*, which produces a strange form of pneumonia. Cell-mediated immune responses are normal and viral infections such as measles and smallpox are readily brought under control. Therapy involves repeated administration of human γ-globulin to maintain adequate concentrations of circulating immunoglobulin.

2. T-cell deficiency

When the thymus fails to develop properly from the third and fourth pharyngeal pouches during embryogenesis, stem cells cannot differentiate to become T-lymphocytes. The 'thymic dependent' areas in lymphoid tissue are sparsely populated but lymphoid follicles with germinal centres and plasma cells are well developed. Cell-mediated immune responses are undetectable and although the infants can deal with common bacterial infections they may be overwhelmed by vaccinia or measles, or by BCG if given by mistake. Humoral antibodies can be elicited but the response is subnormal presumably reflecting the need for the co-operative involvement of T-cells. (The similarity of this condition to neonatal thymectomy and of B-cell deficiency to neonatal bursectomy in the chicken should not go unmentioned.) Treatment by grafting neonatal thymus leads to restoration of immunocompetence but unless graft and donor are well matched, the thymus is ultimately rejected by the ungrateful host cells it has helped to maturity.

3. Stem-cell deficiency

Without proper differentiation of the common lymphoid stem cell, both T- and B-lymphocytes will fail to develop and there will be a severe combined immunodeficiency of cellular and humoral responses. Attempts have been made to treat these patients with grafts of lymphoid stem cells obtained from foetal liver. Temporary restoration of immune function has been reported but where there was a poor histocompatibility match between donor and recipient, the embryonic lymphoid stem cells failed to acquire tolerance to the recipient's antigens and reacted against the host often with a fatal outcome (graft vs. host reaction; chapter 8).

Recognition of immunodeficiencies

Defects in immunoglobulins can be assessed by quantitative estimations using single radial immunodiffusion. Levels of 200 mg/100 ml arbitrarily define the practical lower limit of normal. Selective deficiency in immunoglobulin classes may be established by the same technique. The humoral immune response can be examined by first screening the serum for natural antibodies (A and B isohaemagglutinins, heteroantibody to sheep red cells, bactericidins against *E. coli*) and then attempting to induce active immunization with diphtheria, tetanus, pertussis and killed poliomyelitis—but no live vaccines.

Patients with T-cell deficiency will be hypo- or unreactive in skin tests to such antigens as tuberculin, candida, tricophytin, streptokinase/streptodornase and mumps. Active skin sensitization with dinitrochlorobenzene may be undertaken. The reactivity of peripheral blood mononuclear cells to phytohaemagglutinin is a good indicator of T-lymphocyte reactivity as is also the one-way mixed lymphocyte reaction (see chapter 8).

Further aspects of immunodeficiency disorders

Immunoglobulin deficiency occurs naturally in human infants as the maternal IgG level wanes and may become a serious problem in very premature babies.

IgA deficiency is encountered with relative frequency and these patients often have detectable antibodies to IgA. It is uncertain whether these antibodies prevented development of the IgA system or whether lack of tolerance resulting from an absent IgA system allowed the body to make antibodies to exogenous determinants immunologically related to IgA.

Isolated cases of T-cell deficiency have been reported where the serum contains a lymphocytotoxic antibody which presumably must be selective for T- rather than B-lymphocytes.

Partial deficiencies are more frequently encountered than the extreme cases discussed earlier. Although the majority are still ill defined, two conditions should be mentioned: immunodeficiency with ataxia telangiectasia and immunodeficiency with thrombocytopenia and eczema (Wiskott–Aldrich syndrome). Wiskott–Aldrich is associated with a low IgM and ataxia-telangiectasia a low IgA and IgE. Cell-mediated immunity is depressed in both conditions and it is of interest that about 10 per cent of the patients so far studied have died of malignancies of the lymphoid system or of epithelial tumours. The concomitant lack of IgE with IgA may be partly responsible for the greater susceptibility to upper respiratory infections in ataxia telangiectasia as compared with individuals deficient in IgA alone. Treatment by injection of transfer factor has been attempted and some success reported.

A relatively high incidence of autoantibodies with or without autoimmune disease has been documented in patients with immunodeficiency but the reason for this association is not yet clear.

Secondary immunodeficiency

Immune responsiveness can be depressed non-specifically by many factors. Cell-mediated immunity in particular may be impaired in a state of malnutrition even of the degree which may be encountered in urban areas of the more affluent regions of the world.

Viral infections are not infrequently immunosuppressive and in the case of measles in Man, Newcastle disease in chickens and rinderpest in cattle this has been attributed to a direct cytotoxic effect of virus on the lymphoid cells. In lepromatous leprosy and malarial infection there is evidence for a constraint on immune responsiveness imposed by distortion of the normal lymphoid traffic pathways and additionally, in the latter instance, macrophage function appears to be aberrant. Plasma factors from patients with secondary syphilis which block phytohaemagglutinin transformation of lymphocytes from normal subjects could be responsible for the general reduction in CMI seen in this disease.

Many agents such as X-rays, cytotoxic drugs and corticosteroids, although often used in a non-immunological context, can nonetheless have dire effects on the immune system (p. 195). B-Lymphoproliferative disorders like chronic lymphatic leukaemia, myeloma and Waldenström's macroglobulinaemia are associated with varying degrees of hypo-γ-globulinaemia and impaired antibody responses. Their common infections with pyogenic bacteria contrast with the situation in Hodgkin's disease where the patients display all the hall-marks of T-deficiency—susceptibility to tubercle bacillus, *Brucella cryptococcus* and herpes zoster virus.

Further reading

Godal T., Rees R.J.W. & Lamvik J.O. (1971) Lymphocyte mediated modification of blood derived macrophage function *in vitro*; inhibition of growth of intracellular mycobacteria with lymphokines. *Clin.exp.Immunol.*, **8**, 625.

Gray A.R. (1969) Antigenic variation in trypanosomes. *Bull.World Health Organization*, **41**, 805.

Oakley C.L. (1968) Prophylaxis of microbial diseases. In Gell P.G.H. and Coombs R.R.A. *Clinical Aspects of Immunology,* 2nd ed., p. 1179. Blackwell Scientific Publications, Oxford.

Porter, Ruth & Knight, Julie (1974) *Parasites in the Immunized Host.* Ciba Foundation Symposium, Elsevier, Amsterdam.

Taylor A.E.R. (ed.) (1968) *Immunity to Parasites.* Blackwell Scientific Publications, Oxford.

Wheelock E.F. & Toy S.T. (1973) Participation of lymphocytes in viral infections. *Adv.in Immunology*, **16**, 124.

Wilson G.S. (1967) *The Hazards of Immunization.* Athlone Press, London.

Wright G. (1968) Protective immunity. In Gell P.G.H. & Coombs R.R.A. *Clinical Aspects of Immunology*, 2nd ed., p. 457. Blackwell Scientific Publications, Oxford.

(1971) Primary immunodeficiencies. *W.H.O. Report*, Geneva.

(1973) Cell mediated immunity and resistance to infection. *W.H.O. Technical Report Series,* Geneva.

8 Transplantation

The replacement of diseased organs by a transplant of healthy tissue has long been an objective in medicine but has been frustrated to no mean degree by the unco-operative attempts by the body to reject grafts from other individuals. Before discussing the nature and implications of this rejection phenomenon, it would be helpful to define the terms used for transplants between individuals and species:

Autograft—tissue grafted back onto the original donor.

Isograft—graft between syngeneic individuals (i.e. of identical genetic constitution) such as identical twins or mice of the same pure line strain.

Allograft (old term, homograft)—graft between allogeneic individuals (i.e. members of the same species but different genetic constitution), e.g. man to man and one mouse strain to another.

Xenograft (heterograft)—graft between xenogeneic individuals (i.e. of different species), e.g. pig to man.

It is with the allograft reaction that we have been most concerned although it should one day be possible to use grafts from other species. The most common allografting procedure is probably blood transfusion where the unfortunate consequences of mismatching are well known. Considerable attention has been paid to the rejection of solid grafts such as skin and the sequence of events is worth describing. In mice, for example, the skin homograft settles down and becomes vascularized within a few days. Between three and nine days the circulation gradually diminishes and there is increasing infiltration of the graft bed with lymphocytes and monocytes but very few plasma cells. Necrosis begins to be visible macroscopically and within a day or so the graft is sloughed completely (figure 8.1).

Evidence that rejection is immunological

First and second set reactions

It would be expected if the reaction has an immunological basis, that the second contact with antigen would represent a more

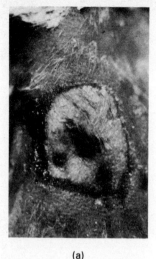 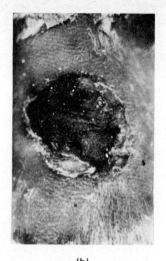

(a)   (b)

FIGURE 8.1. Rejection of CBA skin graft by strain A mouse. (a) 10 days after transplantation; discoloured areas caused by destruction of epithelium and drying of the exposed dermis. (b) 13 days after transplantation; the scabby surface indicates total destruction of the graft. (Courtesy Prof. L. Brent.)

explosive event than the first and indeed the rejection of a second graft from the same donor is much accelerated. The initial vascularization is poor and may not occur at all. There is a very rapid invasion by polymorphonuclear leukocytes and lymphoid cells including plasma cells. Thrombosis and acute cell destruction can be seen by three to four days.

Specificity

Second set rejection is not the fate of all subsequent allografts but only of those derived from the original donor or a related strain. Grafts from unrelated donors are rejected as first set reactions.

Role of the lymphocyte

Neonatally thymectomized animals have difficulty in rejecting skin grafts but their capacity is restored by injection of lymphocytes from a syngeneic normal donor, suggesting that T-cells are implicated. The recipient of lymphoid cells from a donor which has already rejected a graft will give accelerated rejection of a further graft of the same type (figure 8.2) showing that the lymphoid cells are primed and retain memory of the first contact with graft antigens.

182

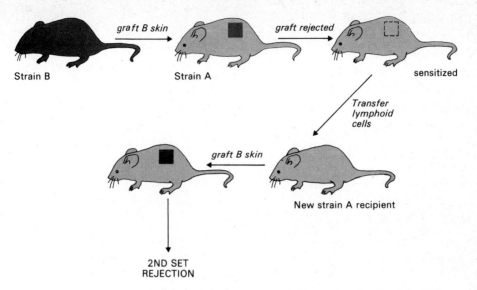

FIGURE 8.2. Transfer of ability to give accelerated graft rejection with lymphoid cells from a sensitized animal.

Production of antibodies

After rejection, humoral antibodies with specificity for the graft donor may be recognized. In the mouse where the erythrocytes carry transplantation antigens, haemagglutination tests become positive; in the human, leucoagglutination is used. A Jerne plaque test using donor strain thymocytes in place of sheep erythrocytes will often demonstrate the presence of antibody-forming cells in the lymphoid tissues of grafted animals.

Transplantation antigens

GENETICS

The specificity of the antigens involved in graft rejection is under genetic control. Genetically identical individuals such as mice of a pure strain or uniovular twins have identical transplantation antigens and grafts can be freely exchanged between them. The Mendelian segregation of the genes controlling these antigens has been revealed by interbreeding experiments between mice of different pure strains. Since these mice breed true within a given strain and always accept grafts from each other, they must be homozygous for the 'transplantation' genes. Consider two such strains A and B with allelic genes

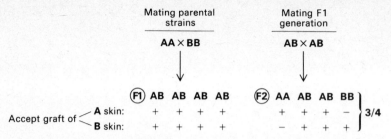

FIGURE 8.3. Inheritance of genes controlling transplantation antigens. A represents a gene expressing the 'A' antigen and B the corresponding allelic gene at the same genetic locus. The pure strains are homozygous for AA and BB respectively. Since the genes are codominant, an animal with an AB genome will express both antigens, become tolerant to them and therefore accept grafts from either A or B donors. The illustration shows that for each gene controlling a transplantation antigen specificity, three-quarters of the F2 generation will accept a graft of parental skin. For n genes the fraction is $(\frac{3}{4})^n$.

differing at one locus. In each case paternal and maternal genes will be identical and they will have a genetic constitution of, say, AA and BB respectively. Crossing strains A and B gives a first familial generation (F1) of constitution AB. These accept grafts from either parent; they must therefore be tolerant to the antigens expressed by both A and B genes and so these genes are codominant, i.e. cells carry both types of transplantation antigen (figure 8.3) as may be shown by immunofluorescent studies. By intercrossing the F1 generation, it will be seen from figure 8.3 that three out of four of the F2 generation accept parental strain grafts. Extending the analysis, if instead of one locus with a pair of allelic genes, there were n loci, the fraction of the F2 generation accepting parental strain grafts would be $(\frac{3}{4})^n$. In this way an estimate of the number of loci controlling transplantation antigens can be made.

In the mouse at least 20 such loci have been established, but of these, one complex locus termed H-2 predominates in the sense that it controls the 'strong' transplantation antigens which provoke intense allograft reactions that are the most difficult to suppress. These antigens are glycoproteins associated largely with the cell surface. Lymphoid cells are rich in H-2 antigens; liver, lung and kidney have moderate amounts, whereas brain and skeletal muscle have very little. The specificity of these histocompatibility antigens probably resides in the amino acid sequence of the protein (although this has not yet been proved) in which case they can be regarded as direct transcriptions of histocompatibility genes. This would account for the large number of specificities which appear to exist.

Although the H-2 locus appeared to be a single entity, it is now seen to be far more complicated and may be broken down into subregions which are separable by genetic recombination (i.e. by chromosomal crossing over between the subregions). Alloantisera obtained by grafting or immunization between different mouse strains define two major subregions H-2K and H-2D (figure 8.4) each representing a major genetic locus (with numerous alleles) which encodes a single 'strong' transplantation antigen. Between them is the Ss subregion which controls a serum protein(s) whose expression is androgen dependent and is linked in some way with the complement system; the insertion of Ss between H-2D and H-2K is considered an evolutionary accident. Between H-2D and Ss lie the very important Ir-1 genes which have been shown to control the immune response to synthetic polypeptides, low doses of ovalbumin, Thy-1^a, thyroid autoantigens and so forth (cf. p. 86). Genetic crossover between genes controlling responsiveness to two different allogeneic myeloma proteins, an IgG and an IgA, suggests that there will prove to be many genes in this region. Genes for graft vs. host reactivity and for lymphocyte activating determinants (see below) also map within these subregions. Overall the major theme which permeates the whole H-2 complex would appear to be recognition of foreignness particularly foreign cells and one may recall the evidence leading to the postulate that the Ir-gene product might in fact be specific T-cell receptor. Note also the Tla gene system close to the H-2D locus, which codes for the TL antigens specific for thymocytes and found on certain thymus leukaemia cells. The H-2 antigens themselves may well prove to subserve some primitive cellular recognition system. *Hh* factors controlled by genes in the same region, confer resistance to bone marrow grafts in non-syngeneic irradiated recipients, e.g. F1 into parent (presumably reflecting non-codominant expression of Hh genes). Other genes mapping near H-2K are Rgv-1 which confers resistance to Gross leukaemia virus by suppressing the expression of virus associated antigen, and Hom-1 which influences the level of testosterone and testosterone-binding protein. Because all these genes are linked together on a single chromosome (haplotype) they will appear to segregate as a single Mendelian trait, the complexity only being revealed by crossing over and recombination.

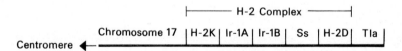

FIGURE 8.4 Subregions of the H-2 gene complex. The H-2K product provokes a more powerful transplantation reaction than H-2D. The Ir-IA subregion includes one series of genes controlling immune responsiveness, H-2I influencing the expression of a further moderately powerful transplantation antigen, Lad-1 concerned with surface products which lead to lymphocyte activation (lymphocyte activating determinants; also called lymphocyte determined, LD, specificities by Bach) in the mixed lymphocyte reaction (see below) and Gvh-1 which controls the determinants responsible for graft-versus-host reactivity (also explained below). Single gene products may prove to be responsible for 2 or more of these properties. The Ir-IB subregion embraces Ir-IB, Lad-2 and Gvh-2 genes. The Ss subregion includes the Ss-Slp loci coding for sex-linked serum protein(s) possible related to complement levels.

Serologically defined determinants

In man, as in the mouse, there is also one dominant group of antigens which provokes strong reactions—the HL-A system—which represents the counterpart of the H-2 system. In addition the ABO group provides strong transplantation antigens.

Because humans cannot be manipulated in the same manner as mice it proved much harder to analyse the HL-A system. Polyspecific antisera were obtained from patients receiving multiple transfusions of whole blood, individuals deliberately immunized with skin grafts or leukocyte injections, patients who had rejected an organ graft and multigravidas who often become immunized with foetal antigens with specificities defined by paternally derived genes absent from the mother's genome. Approximately 100 such sera were tested for lymphocyte agglutination reactions against panels of 50 to several hundred randomly selected donors. The results obtained with each serum were compared with those obtained with every other serum by computer analysis and this enabled van Rood to classify the sera into a relatively small number of groups such that if *all* sera in one group consistently react with the cells of *one* individual, they may be considered to indicate a single specificity.

We now use complement-mediated cytotoxic tests with lymphocytes or platelets as targets to establish tissue type and the procedure has been greatly simplified by the availability of reference sera which are operationally mono-specific. This serological approach combined with the study of family inheritance has defined at least two major subloci of the HL-A system (cf. H-2K and H-2D in the mouse) and probably a third so far largely unexplored. The antigens numbered HL-A1, 2, 3, 9, 10, 11 and 28 are negatively associated with each other in population studies, no individual has more than two of these specificities and not more than one is transmitted to each offspring; they therefore form an allelic series referred to as the first sublocus of the HL-A system. HL-A5, 7, 8, 12, 13, 14, 17 and 27 constitute a second sublocus present on the same chromosome as the first. Thus, an individual heterozygous at each locus must express four major HL-A specificities, two from maternally derived and two from the paternally derived chromosomes (figure 8.5).

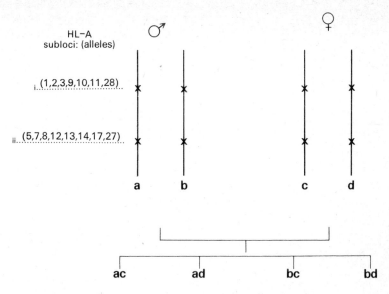

HL-A
subloci: (alleles)

i. (1,2,3,9,10,11,28)

ii. (5,7,8,12,13,14,17,27)

a   b   c   d

ac   ad   bc   bd

FIGURE 8.5. Inheritance of HL-A specificities. Each offspring has a paternal and a maternal chromosome each bearing two HL-A alleles. Since there are several possible alleles at each locus, the probability of a random pair from the general population having identical HL-A specificities is low. The same holds for parent-offspring pairings. However there is a 1:4 change that two siblings will be identical in this respect because each pair of specificities on a single chromosome (haplotype) form a linkage group which will be inherited *en bloc*.

Lymphocyte activating determinants

When lymphocytes from genetically dissimilar subjects are cultured together, a *mixed lymphocyte reaction* (MLR) involving blast cell transformation and mitosis occurs, each population of lymphocytes reacting against 'foreign' determinants in the other population. These surface lymphocyte activating determinants (Lad) are not identical with the serologically defined HL-A specificities although the genes which code for them map very closely to the HL-A loci so that the HL-A and Lad genes on a given chromosome tend to be inherited as a single linkage group (cf. figure 8.4). Thus HL-A compatible siblings nearly always fail to react against each other in mixed lymphocyte reactions. The chance of Lad being identical on lymphocytes from unrelated donors matched for HL-A will be lower to the extent that Lad and HL-A genes drift apart in the population. Coming to HL-A incompatible unrelated donors, it appears that the chance of finding one pair which fail to react against each other in the MLR must be less, possibly much less, than 1:500.

The relevance of Lad to the provocation of transplantation rejection has been brought into some focus by the discovery of the phenomenon of *cell mediated lympholysis* (CML) which was developed as a possible test for histoincompatibility. The principle is illustrated in figure 8.6. In short, if lymphocytes from donor B react against A in one-way mixed lymphocyte culture because of differences in Lad, the transformed lymphoblasts are cytotoxic for A cells provided there are HL-A incompatibilities between them. With unrelated but HL-A matched individuals, the transformed cells resulting from the MLR will not be cytotoxic for the other member of the pair. The importance of these phenomena for graft survival has yet to be evaluated.

Graft vs. host (g.v.h.) reaction

When competent lymphoid cells are transferred from a donor to a recipient which is incapable of rejecting them, the grafted cells survive and have time to recognize the host antigens and react immunologically against them. Instead of the normal transplantation reaction of host against graft, we have the reverse, the

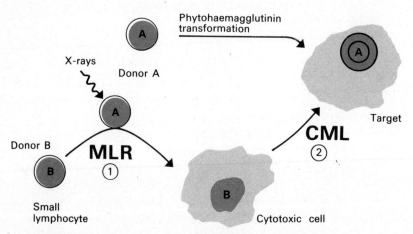

FIGURE 8.6. Cell mediated lympholysis. *Stage (1)—Mixed lymphocyte reaction* indicating differences in Lad: B's lymphocytes divide and transform into killer cells on recognizing Lad on A but A's lymphocytes cannot react reciprocally since they have been blocked by X-irradiation. Meanwhile a separate sample of A's lymphocytes are transformed into blasts with PHA and labelled with radioactive chromium; these will act as targets for stage 2 and are more vulnerable than small lymphocytes.
   Stage (2)—Cytotoxic reaction depending on HL-A differences: an excess of transformed B lymphoblasts will be cytotoxic for labelled A target cells as evidenced by chromium release.

188

so-called graft vs. host reaction. In the young rodent there can be inhibition of growth (runting), spleen enlargement and haemolytic anaemia (due to production of red cell antibodies). In the human, fever, anaemia, weight loss, rash, diarrhoea and splenomegaly are observed. The 'stronger' the transplantation antigen difference, the more severe the reaction. Where donor and recipient differ at HL-A or H-2 loci, the reaction can be fatal.

Two possible situations leading to g.v.h. reactions are illustrated in figure 8.7. In the human this may arise in immunologically anergic subjects receiving bone marrow grafts, e.g. for combined immunodeficiency (p. 177), for red cell aplasia after radiation accidents or as a possible form of cancer therapy. Competent lymphoid cells in blood or present in grafted organs given to immunosuppressed patients may give g.v.h. reactions; so could maternal cells which adventitiously cross the placenta, although in this case there is as yet no evidence of diseases caused by such a mechanism in the human. In the rare cases where autoantibodies to lymphoid cells arise this may be looked upon as a special example of the g.v.h. reaction.

Rejection mechanisms

LYMPHOCYTE-MEDIATED REJECTION

A great deal of the work on allograft rejection has involved transplants of skin or solid tumours because their fate is relatively easy to follow. In these cases there is little support for the

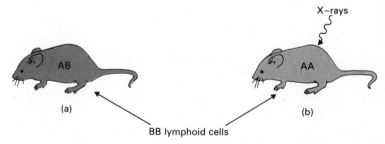

FIGURE 8.7. Graft vs. host reaction. When competent lymphoid cells are inoculated into a host incapable of reacting against them, the grafted cells are free to react against the antigens on the host's cells which they recognize as foreign. The ensuing reaction may be fatal. Two of many possible situations are illustrated: (a) the hybrid AB receives cells from one parent (BB) which are tolerated but react against the A antigen on host cells (b) an X-irradiated AA recipient restored immunologically with BB cells cannot react against the graft and a g.v.h. reaction will result.

view that humoral antibodies are instrumental in destruction of the graft although as we shall see later this is not necessarily so with transplants of other organs such as the kidney. Whereas passive transfer of *serum* from an animal which has rejected a skin allograft cannot usually accelerate the rejection of a similar graft on the recipient animal, injection of *lymphoid cells* (particularly recirculating small lymphocytes) is effective in shortening graft survival (cf. figure 8.2). Tissue culture studies have shown that such lymphoid cells taken from animals sensitized by a graft which they have rejected are able to kill target cells possessing the same transplantation antigens as the original graft. The sensitized lymphocytes recognize the target cells through specific surface receptors and this combination with antigen leads to surface membrane changes responsible for the cytotoxic potential of the lymphocytes (through the activation of membrane-bound C8 ?).

A primary role of lymphoid cells in first set rejection would be consistent with the histology of the early reaction showing infiltration by mononuclear cells with very few polymorphs or plasma cells (figure 8.8). The dramatic effect of neonatal thymectomy in prolonging skin transplants, as mentioned earlier, and the long survival of grafts on children with thymic deficiencies implicate the T-lymphocytes in these reactions. In the chicken, homograft rejection and g.v.h. reactivity are influenced by neonatal thymectomy but not bursectomy. More direct evidence has come from *in vitro* studies showing that the sensitized mouse lymphocytes responsible for killing target graft cells in tissue culture bear the θ marker on their surface (see p. 57) and are therefore T-lymphocytes.

Lymphoid cells sensitized to a graft can release macrophage migration inhibition factor (MIF; see p. 150) when confronted with the appropriate histocompatibility antigens and it is possible that this test will give an early indication of sensitization in a grafted individual.

THE ROLE OF HUMORAL ANTIBODY

It has long been recognized that isolated allogeneic cells such as lymphocytes can be destroyed by cytotoxic (type II) reactions involving humoral antibody. However, although earlier experience with skin and solid tumour-grafts suggested that they were not readily susceptible to the action of cytotoxic antibodies, it is now clear that this does not hold for all types of organ transplants. Consideration of the different ways in which kidney allografts can be rejected illustrates the point:

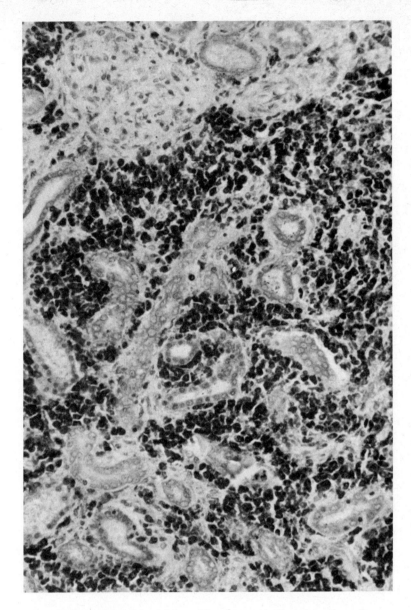

FIGURE 8.8. Acute early rejection of human renal allograft 10 days after transplantation showing dense cellular infiltration of tubules by mononuclear cells. (Courtesy Prof. K. Porter.)

(a) *Hyperacute rejection* within minutes of transplantation, characterized by sludging of red cells and microthrombi in the glomeruli, occurs in individuals with pre-existing humoral antibodies—either due to blood group incompatibility or presensitization through blood transfusion.

(b) *Acute early rejection* occurring up to 10 days or so after transplantation is characterized by dense cellular infiltration (figure 8.8) and rupture of peritubular capillaries and appears to be a cell-mediated hypersensitivity reaction involving T-lymphocytes.

(c) *Acute late rejection*, which occurs from 11 days onwards in patients suppressed with prednisone and azathioprine, is

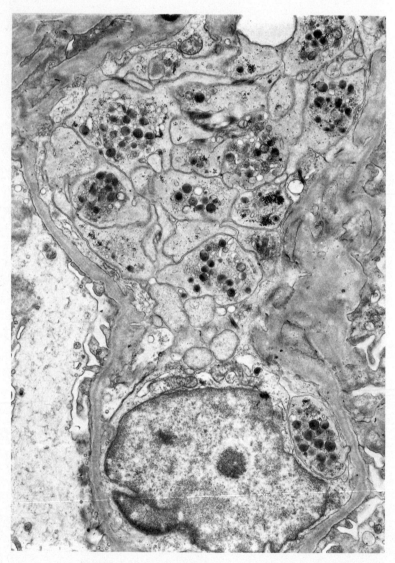

FIGURE 8.9. Acute late rejection of human renal allograft showing platelet aggregation in a glomerular capillary induced by deposition of antibody on the vessel wall. (Courtesy Prof. K. Porter.)

probably caused by the binding of immunoglobulin (presumably antibody) and complement to the arterioles and glomerular capillaries where they can be visualized by immunofluorescent techniques. These immunoglobulin deposits on the vessel walls induce platelet aggregation in the glomerular capillaries leading to acute renal shutdown (figure 8.9).

(d) *Insidious and late* rejection associated with subendothelial deposits of immunoglobulin and C3 on the glomerular basement membranes which may sometimes be an expression of an underlying immune complex disorder (originally necessitating the transplant) or possibly complex formation with soluble antigens derived from the grafted kidney.

In addition to these mechanisms Perlmann has found that humoral antibody coating a target cell makes it susceptible to cytotoxic attack by normal unsensitized (K) lymphoid cells. This emphasizes the complexity of the action and interaction of cellular and humoral factors in graft rejection and other tissue hypersensitivities (figure 8.10).

There are also circumstances when antibodies may actually *protect* a graft from destruction and this important phenomenon of *enhancement* will be considered further below.

Prevention of graft rejection

TISSUE MATCHING

Based upon experience of matching blood for transfusion and of transplantation between mice of similar specificities it could reasonably be expected that the chances of rejection in the human would be minimized by matching donor and recipient at the HL-A locus. Notwithstanding the complications which may arise from lymphocyte activating determinants (ascertained from mixed lymphocyte reactions) in unrelated but HL-A identical donors in the case of human kidney transplantation, it is clear that the closer the match, the better the survival of the graft (figure 8.11). The results with kidneys taken from unrelated cadavers show the same trend with respect to HL-A matching but overall survival is less satisfactory than with sibling material probably as a consequence of deterioration in the organ before grafting.

Because of the many thousands of different HL-A phenotypes possible (figure 8.5), it is usual to work with a large pool of potential recipients on a continental basis so that when graft material becomes available the best possible match can be

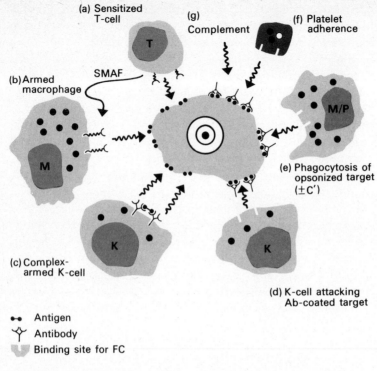

(a) Sensitized T-cell

(g) Complement

(f) Platelet adherence

(b) Armed macrophage

SMAF

(e) Phagocytosis of opsonized target (±C′)

(c) Complex-armed K-cell

(d) K-cell attacking Ab-coated target

•• Antigen
Y Antibody
⊔ Binding site for FC

FIGURE 8.10. Mechanisms of target cell destruction. (a) Direct killing by sensitized T cells binding through specific surface receptors. In addition a non-specific soluble toxin and specific macrophage arming factor (SMAF—perhaps T-cell receptor often complexed with antigen; cf p. 150) are released. (b) Killing by SMAF-armed macrophages. (c) Specific killing by immune-complex-armed K-cell which recognizes target through free antibody valencies in the complex. (d) Attack by K-cell on antibody-coated target cell (in a–d the killing is extra-cellular). (e) Phagocytosis of target coated with antibody (heightened by bound C3). (f) Sticking of platelets to antibody bound to surface of graft vascular endothelium leading to formation of microthrombi. (g) Complement mediated cytoxicity.

made. The position will be improved when the pool of available organs can be increased through the development of long-term tissue storage banks but techniques are not good enough for this at present except in the case of bone marrow cells which can be kept viable even after freezing and thawing. With a paired organ such as the kidney, living donors may be used; siblings provide the best chance of a good match (cf. figure 8.5). However, the use of living donors poses difficult ethical problems and the objective must be to perfect the use of cadaver material (? or animal organs—or mechanical substitutes!).

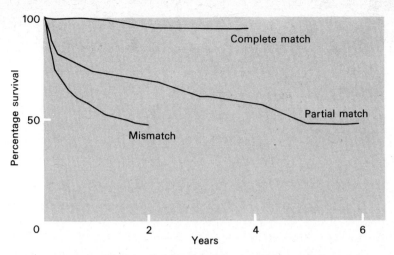

FIGURE 8.11. Survival of kidney transplants in relation to degree of HL-A matching. Complete match (siblings) = all HL-A antigens identical; partial match (siblings and parent to child) = only antigens on one chromosome (haplotype) identical; mismatch (unrelated) = all HL-A antigens different. (Data taken from J. Dausset & J. Hors, *Transpl. Proc.* 1973, **V**, 223).

GENERAL IMMUNOSUPPRESSION

Graft rejection can be held at bay by the use of agents which non-specifically interfere with the induction or expression of the immune response. Because these agents are non-specific, patients on immunosuppressive therapy may be particularly susceptible to infections; they are also more prone to develop cancer.

Lymphoid cell ablation

Thymectomy, splenectomy and lymphadenectomy in adult recipients do not appear to help. Whole-body irradiation is too drastic although extra-corporeal irradiation of blood and thoracic duct cannulation have proved beneficial.

Immunosuppressive drugs

The development of an immunological response requires the active proliferation of a relatively small number of antigen-sensitive lymphocytes to give a population of sensitized cells large enough to be effective. Many of the immunosuppressive drugs now employed were first used in cancer chemotherapy because of their toxicity to dividing cells. Aside from the complications of blanket immunosuppression mentioned above, these antimitotic drugs are especially toxic for cells of the bone marrow and small intestine and must therefore be used with great care.

Perhaps the most commonly used drug in this field is *azathioprine* which is broken down in the body first to 6-mercaptopurine and then converted to the active agent, the ribotide. Because of the similarity in shape (figure 8.12), this competes with inosinic acid for enzymes concerned in the synthesis of guanylic and adenylic acids; it also inhibits the synthesis of 5-phosphoribosylamine, a precursor of inosinic acid, by a feedback mechanism. The net result is inhibition of nucleic acid synthesis. Another drug, methotrexate, through its action as a folic acid antagonist also inhibits synthesis of nucleic acid. The N-mustard derivative cyclophosphamide probably attacks DNA by alkylation and cross-linking so preventing correct duplication during cell division. These agents appear to exert their damaging effects on cells during mitosis and for this reason are most powerful when administered after presentation of antigen at a time when the antigen-sensitive cells are dividing.

Steroids such as prednisone intervene at many points in the immune response but are outstandingly potent as anti-inflammatory drugs inhibiting the effector mechanisms of graft rejection. Azathioprine is also known to inhibit inflammation, and many think that it acts more as an anti-inflammatory drug than an immunosuppressive agent at the doses used in man where it is commonly employed in combination with prednisone.

Antilymphocyte globulin (ALG)

There has been a considerable resurgence of interest in the immunosuppressive properties of heterologous anti-lymphocyte sera. To prepare anti-human lymphocyte serum horses are

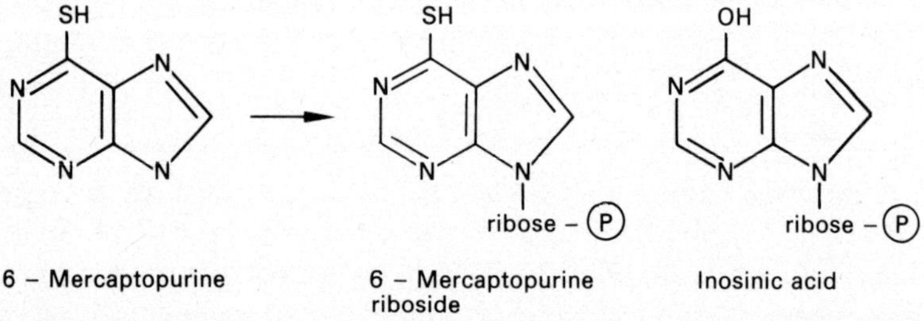

6 – Mercaptopurine   6 – Mercaptopurine riboside   Inosinic acid

FIGURE 8.12. Metabolic conversion of azathioprine through 6-mercaptopurine to the ribotide: similarity to inosinic acid with which it competes.

immunized with human thymocytes or thoracic duct lymphocytes, serum collected and absorbed with red cells to remove agglutinins; finally a globulin fraction is isolated.

Assessment of potency. Immunosuppressive activity of different ALG preparations *in vivo* has been evaluated by the ability to prolong skin homografts in monkeys and chimpanzees. Limited studies of this kind in man have also shown immunosuppressive effects.

In vitro, ALG can cause lymphoagglutination, complement-mediated killing of lymphocytes and with some preparations, blast-cell transformation. A test with good predictive value for *in vitro* potency involves complement-mediated inhibition by ALG of background rosette formation between human peripheral lymphocytes and sheep erythrocytes. The basis of the test appears to be steric hindrance of red cell binding to the lymphocyte surface by complement components C1 and C4 fixed to the ALG–lymphocyte complex.

Lymphocytes coated with ALG will adhere 'opsonically' to macrophages in monolayer culture and this adherence reaction can be made much more sensitive by addition of complement since there are receptors on the macrophage for both Fcγ (the Fc part of IgG) and C3 following their involvement in an antigen–antibody reaction (see 162). The titre of an ALG in such a C-dependent immune adherence reaction is a good guide to its immunosuppressive action *in vivo* in mice and to a lesser extent in primates.

Mode of action. In mice and rats, ALG can dramatically prolong the life of skin homografts. If given to an animal which has been sensitized by graft rejection, it can erase the memory of the primary contact with antigen and if challenged some time afterwards with a second graft from the same donor, there will be first, not second, set rejection as though the animal were immunologically 'virgin' with respect to those histocompatibility antigens. Graft vs. host reactions and humoral antibody responses involving T-cell co-operation are also especially sensitive to ALG treatment, suggesting that the T-lymphocyte is the primary target. In accord with this view:

(i) ALG depletes the 'thymus dependent' areas of lymphoid tissue, the lymphocytes being replaced by histiocytic cells, and

(ii) after ALG there is a sharp fall in the ability of peripheral lymphocytes to give blast-cell transformation in response to PHA (largely a characteristic of T-lymphocytes; p. 153). The return of PHA responsiveness is retarded by thymectomy

197

(figure 8.13) pointing up the significance of T-cell maturation for recovery from the ALG lesion.

The T-cell may be more vulnerable to ALG action because of antigens not possessed by B-cells, or a greater surface concentration of common antigens; furthermore the recirculating T-cell when present in the blood is readily accessible to ALG whereas the B-cells in lymphoid tissue tend to remain where they are.

There are probably several mechanisms which could operate to inhibit T-lymphocyte function (figure 8.14):

(a) at relatively high ALG concentrations the cells would be killed by a complement mediated cytotoxic reaction;

(b) at much lower concentrations enough C3 would be bound to give an immune adherence to macrophages (and red cells in primates) which would result in lymphocyte removal by phagocytosis;

(c) at the same or even lower concentrations, enough C1 and C4 might be bound to blindfold the lymphocyte and prevent it from recognizing antigen;

(d) ALG could inhibit vital membrane changes occurring as a result of antigen stimulation or might contain antibodies able

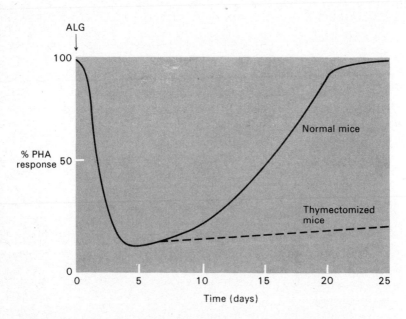

FIGURE 8.13. Effect of injected anti-lymphocyte globulin on mitotic response of peripheral mouse lymphocytes to phytohaemagglutinin (PHA). Results are expressed as a percentage of the pretreatment response. Mice recover to normal values by approximately day 20 but this recovery is not seen in thymectomized animals (from Tursi A. *et al. Immunology* 1969, **17**, 801).

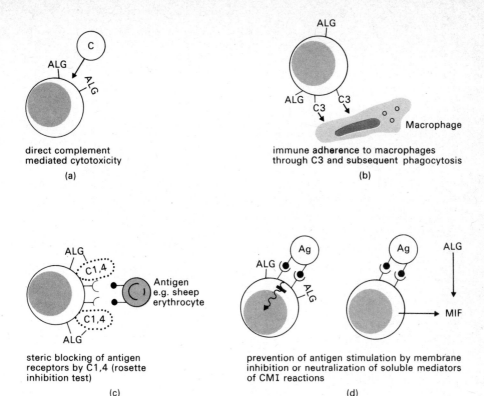

direct complement
mediated cytotoxicity

(a)

immune adherence to macrophages
through C3 and subsequent phagocytosis

(b)

steric blocking of antigen
receptors by C1,4 (rosette
inhibition test)

(c)

prevention of antigen stimulation by membrane
inhibition or neutralization of soluble mediators
of CMI reactions

(d)

FIGURE 8.14. Possible modes of action of anti-lymphocyte globulin (ALG).

to neutralize some of the soluble factors concerned in cell-mediated immunity.

Clinical use. ALG produces pain at the site of intramuscular injection and the intravenous route carries the risk of kidney damage through immune complex formation with the horse IgG. For prolonged administration of ALG it would seem desirable to induce tolerance to horse IgG and there are indications that this is possible using deaggregated material. The concentrations of ALG used in the human are much lower than those normally produced in laboratory animals and it is by no means clear that the doses normally employed in clinical practice are in fact immunosuppressive or anti-inflammatory. It is difficult to assess the therapeutic benefit attributable to ALG but at the present time the 'impressions' of most clinicians are favourable. ALG is of benefit in bone marrow transplants particularly in the elimination of immunocompetent cells from the graft; it may well be of value in the treatment of certain rejection crises and perhaps in the induction of tolerance.

Immunological tolerance

If the disadvantages of blanket immunosuppression are to be avoided, we must aim at knocking out only the reactivity of the host to the antigens of the graft leaving the remainder of the immunological apparatus intact. One approach is through the induction of tolerance in the patient. Purified histocompatibility antigens are slowly becoming available and it is to be hoped that we can so manipulate the patient that continued low doses of antigen possibly combined with ALG or other immuno-suppressive treatment will lead to a specific hyporesponsive state. Attempts are also being made to establish tolerance by injection of an (idiotypic) antiserum considered to be specific for those T-cell receptors in the host which recognize donor transplantation antigens.

Enhancement

There is another possible solution which may be easier to achieve and that is deliberate immunization with these anti-gens to evoke antibodies which protect rather than destroy the graft. Such *enhancing* antibodies have long been recognized as being responsible for the prolonged survival of tumour allo-grafts under appropriate circumstances, and the phenomenon can be reproduced *in vitro* where the killing of target cells by sensitized lymphocytes from an H-2 incompatible mouse is inhibited by addition of antibodies directed against the H-2 antigens of the target. Presumably the antibodies combine with the surface antigens of the target cells which are then no longer accessible to the receptors on the aggressor lymphocytes. The antibodies must, of course, combine with the target cell in a manner which avoids the activation of complement or indeed of non-specific K aggressor cells (p. 136). In the case of com-plement at least, this would occur if the determinants on the surface were too far apart to allow the Fc portions of adjacent antibodies to interact and bind complement (cf. p. 120) and might also be insufficient to allow effective interaction with K-cells; alternatively if the antigenic determinants were close together, no activation of C1 or of K-cells would be possible if there were a preponderance of antibodies belonging to in-appropriate immunoglobulin classes (figure 8.15). The situa-tion is quite different when cytotoxicity is mediated by complex-armed K-cells (cf. figure 8.10) since in order to

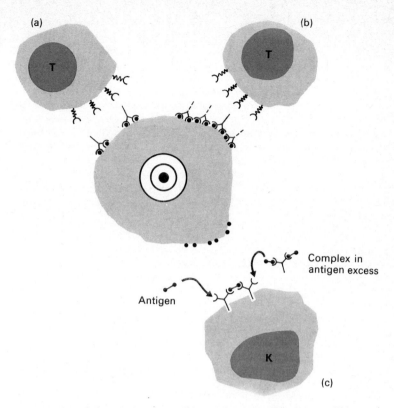

(a)

(b)

(c)

Complex in
antigen excess

Antigen

FIGURE 8.15. Enhancement: possible mechanisms. The target cell is
protected from agressor cell attack by antibody *masking* the surface
antigens, or by antigen, frequently in the form of antigen excess complexes,
blocking the effector cell. The masking antibody should not fix complement
(otherwise the cell could be killed by this alone) and this would happen
(a) if the antigen has a low surface density and the antibody Fc regions
are not adjacent or (b) if non-complement fixing antibodies ($\rangle$--)
predominated. Neither should the antibodies belong mainly to classes
which allow K-cell binding to occur. Where the aggressor is a K-cell
armed with antigen-antibody complexes (c) the spare antibody valencies
which allow binding to the target can be blocked by free or complexed
antigen present in the serum in the manner shown.

protect the grafted cell it is necessary to block the spare antibody valencies on the K-cell surface complex and this can be
effected by soluble antigen, either free or in complexes formed
in antigen excess.

Successful enhancement of kidney and bone-marrow grafts
have been reported in isolated instances and one supposes this
will inevitably be extended. There are indications that serum
enhancing factors may inhibit tumour destruction by cell-
mediated mechanisms in some cancer patients as will be discussed later.

The controversial suggestion has been made that the phenomenon of immunological tolerance to transplantation antigens (p. 76) may be explained in terms of enhancement. This stems from the finding that the lymphoid cells of a CBA animal although tolerant to and bearing a skin graft of A, may nonetheless be capable of inhibiting the growth of A strain cells in culture as do cells from an immunized mouse; however serum from these animals blocks the *in vitro* effect and it is postulated that this serum factor is protecting the graft. The explanation might run on the following lines. T-cells are more readily tolerized than B and it may be that the tolerance-inducing regimen does truly tolerize T cells (which are therefore unable to reject the skin graft) but not all B-cells. These B cells make antibody to graft antigens which arm K-cells and make them effective in the microculture test against A cells; this reaction is blocked by serum factors (antigen or complexes). That the T-cells are tolerant is shown by their loss of ability to give graft vs. host reactions.

Clinical experience in grafting

Privileged sites

Corneal grafts survive without the need for immunosuppression. Because they are avascular they do not sensitize the recipient although they become cloudy if the individual has been presensitized. Grafts of cartilage are successful in the same way but an additional factor is the protection afforded the chondrocytes by the matrix.

Kidney

Over 3,000 kidneys have been transplanted and with improvement in patient management there is a high survival rate (figure 8.11). Patients are partially immunosuppressed at the time of transplantation because uraemia causes a degree of immunological anergy. If kidney function is poor during a rejection crisis renal dialysis can be used. When transplantation is performed because of immune complex induced glomerulonephritis, the usual immuno-suppressive regimen of azathioprine and prednisone may help to prevent a similar lesion developing in the grafted kidney. Patients with glomerular basement membrane antibodies (e.g. Goodpasture's syndrome) are likely to destroy their renal transplants.

Heart

Something like 40–50% of transplanted patients survive by one year. The results have not been as good as with kidney grafting but special factors should be taken into account. The recipient patients were in irreversible cardiac failure with wasting and advanced secondary changes of passive congestion and the clinical urgency made it difficult to find well-matched donor organs. Aside from the rejection problem it is likely that the number of patients who would benefit from cardiac replacement is much greater than the number dying with adequately healthy hearts. More attention will have to be given to the possibility of xenogeneic grafts and mechanical substitutes.

Liver

Survival rates for orthotopic liver grafts are broadly in line with those receiving heart transplants. Three-quarters of the patients transplanted for hepatic cancer have had recurrence of their tumour within one year.

Experience with liver grafting between pigs revealed an unexpected finding. Many of the animals retained the grafted organs in a healthy state for many months without any form of immunosuppression. The transplanted liver represented a large antigen pool which induced a state of unresponsiveness to grafts of skin or kidney from the same donor. The mechanism is not clear but may involve true tolerance or enhancement. There is as yet no evidence that this highly desirable state can be established by a hepatic transplant in man.

Lymphoreticular tissue

Certain immunodeficiency disorders and some forms of anaemia are obvious candidates for treatment with lymphoid stem cells and in the future we may expect further attempts to transfer immunocompetent cells as an approach to the treatment of cancer. Successful results with bone marrow (and immunocompetent cell) transfers require highly compatible donors if fatal graft vs. host reactions are to be avoided, and here siblings offer the best chance of finding a matched donor (figure 8.5).

The question may be asked, why do unmatched foetal liver or bone marrow cells which are presumed to be immunologically immature, not become tolerant to the host antigens as they develop, as might be expected from the experiments on tolerance induction by injection of the newborn described in chapter 3? It appears that there are many histocompatibility antigen specificities involved in most cases and it is difficult for the injected cells to induce tolerance to *all* specificities.

Other organs

It is to be expected that improvement in techniques of control of the rejection process will encourage transplantation in several other areas. Not, of course, in most cases of endocrine disorders where exogenous replacement therapy is available, but one looks forward to the successful transplantation of lungs, of skin for lethal burns, and even of bones and joints.

The cancer cell and the allograft reaction

The ability to reject transplants of tissue may be traced back a long way down the evolutionary tree—back even as far as the annelid worms. Obviously this faculty did not develop in order to thwart the transplantation surgeon; it must confer survival advantage on the host. One possibility, suggested by Lewis Thomas, was that the immunological system policed the body cells, keeping an eye open for altered cells which might become neoplastic. For this *immunological surveillance* mechanism to operate, cancer cells must display a new surface antigen which can be recognized by the lymphoid cells and indeed they do.

TUMOUR SURFACE ANTIGENS

These antigens can be considered under four main headings:
   (a) *Virally controlled*. Cells infected with oncogenic viruses display a new transplantation antigen on their surface which is characteristic of the infecting virus. All tumours induced by a given virus carry the same surface antigen irrespective of their morphological characteristics, so that immunization with one tumour confers resistance to subsequent challenge with any other syngeneic tumour induced by the same virus.
   (b) *Embryonic*. Tumours derived from the same cell type often express a common differentiation antigen also present on embryonic cells (so-called oncofoetal antigens). Examples would be α-foetoprotein in hepatic carcinoma and carcino-embryonic antigen (CEA) in cancer of the intestine.
   (c) *Division*. Antigens on the cell surface may change during cell division. For example, Thomas found that the density of surface sugar determinants with blood group H specificity fell as murine mastocytoma cells moved into the G_1 phase of the division cycle while reciprocally, group B determinants increased; it was postulated that the continued expression of this latter component was related to a commitment to further division. Tumour cell lines of B-lymphocyte derivation display a surface antigen absent from resting B lymphocytes which might therefore have been labelled a tumour specific antigen had not activated B-cell blasts also been shown to express it.

The oncofoetal antigens may sometimes merely represent division antigens.

(d) *Idiotypic*. Tumours induced by chemical agents, benzopyrene for example, also possess specific transplantation antigens. However, they differ from virally induced neoplasms in that each tumour produced by a given chemical carcinogen has its own individual idiotypic antigen; even when a carcinogen produces two different primary tumours in the same animal, they do not exhibit the same antigenic specificities.

Burnet has looked at this in a novel way. The carcinogen could have induced the synthesis of a new antigen (Lamarckian viewpoint), in which case it is difficult to see why each tumour expresses an individual antigen unless each represents the activation of a different oncogenic virus or the product of a new mutation; or the antigen pre-existed on just a few cells and only became demonstrable through multiplication of these cells (a selective Darwinian hypothesis). Taking the latter approach, Burnet postulated that regions on certain transplantation antigens might be subject to a high degree of mutation generating a wide diversity of specificities. This may be looked upon as complementary to the generation of antibody diversity in lymphoid cells which are therefore potentially capable of recognizing the newly formed transplantation antigen specificities. They do not do so normally because only very few cells have each antigen specifity and these are insufficient to evoke an immune response—or tolerance. However, if a cell is selected by the carcinogen and divides to form a large clone of neoplastic cells, the clonal antigen can now be recognized (by us as a tumour specific antigen) and the immunological surveillance mechanism should be activated.

IMMUNE RESPONSE TO TUMOURS

These tumour antigens can provoke a variety of immune responses in experimental animals which frequently lead to resistance against tumour growth. Circulating antibody can clearly be cytotoxic for tumours which persist in the form of isolated cells, but K- and T-cells would seem to be needed for the onslaught on a solid tumour. A number of *in vitro* tests have been developed to evaluate the tumour-specific immune response. The release of radioactive chromium from the labelled tumour by lymphoid cells from resistant animals is usually ascribable to T-lymphocyte reactivity. Tests involving the ability of the animal's leucocytes to inhibit the growth of tumour cells in microcultures (colony inhibition, microcytotoxicity, cytostasis tests) are likely to reflect the activity of K-cells. When serum from animals in which the tumour is *regressing* is added to such a micro-cytotoxicity system it fails to influence the outcome of the test, but serum from animals with *progressive* tumours contains enhancing or blocking factors which can abrogate the inhibitory effect of the cells on the tumour (Hellstrom's). It would seem plausible to suggest that these blocking agents could in fact protect the tumour from cellular attack *in vivo*. The blocking factors often prove to be either free antigen or complexes formed in antigen excess (cf. p. 201 and figure 8.15) and can be eliminated by stimulating antibody formation in the tumour-bearing animal (e.g. by B.C.G. infection) so that the balance between antigen and antibody is tipped towards the latter giving complexes which are no longer inhibitory.

We have evidence that immunological processes are operative in human cancer. For example, cytotoxic antibodies have been found in the sera of a proportion of patients with malignant melanoma and these apparently act to prevent metastasis of the tumour. The presence of lymphoid reaction in the draining nodes and infiltration of the tumour with mononuclear inflammatory cells is a good prognostic sign in cancer of the breast; early reports indicate that extracts of these tumours cause specific inhibition of the migration of autologous leukocytes *in vitro* (MIF test). Burkitt lymphoma patients can develop serum antibodies which react with antigens on cells of their own and other Burkitt tumours which are controlled by a herpes-like organism, the Epstein-Barr (EB) virus. Lymphoid cells from subjects with neuroblastoma are sometimes cytotoxic for (or prevent division of) cells from their own tumour and from other neuroblastomas *in vitro*. Similar findings have been reported with cancer of the bladder, suggesting that a given type of tumour may always carry a characteristic antigen. A hint of an oncogenic virus? The expression of a degree of dedifferentiation linked with the neoplastic change? Or perhaps an onco-foetal or division antigen? At the time of writing the indications are that this cytotoxic activity may frequently depend upon K-cells and not necessarily on T-lymphocytes as we have so readily assumed in the past. Of considerable interest is the finding of blocking factors in the serum of a proportion of these patients presumably analogous to those described in the tumour-bearing animals.

IMMUNOTHERAPY

When cell-mediated immunity is depressed by long-term treatment with immunosuppressive drugs and anti-lymphocyte serum, there is a significantly increased tendency to develop cancer. If we examine non-debilitated cancer patients there is a relative depression in CMI reactivity assessed by PHA and mixed lymphocyte reactions of peripheral blood and the development of contact hypersensitivity to dinitrochloro-benzene applied to the skin.

There could be a relationship between the increased inci-dence of cancer in old age and the gradual fall off in CMI. Thinking along these lines and taking into account the older view that enhancement worked only by antibody masking tumour antigens, it is not surprising that the oversimplistic notion was entertained that in cancer we should activate CMI and depress humoral antibody production whereas in the field of transplantation where the objectives are completely reversed the aim should be to avoid CMI and stimulate enhancing anti-body. Alas, the reader knows that we must inject into the overall equation armed macrophages, K-cells, complexes which arm K-cells, serum complexes which block armed K-cells and antibody which can 'unblock' this effect let alone the affinities and immunoglobulin classes of the antibodies we are stimulat-ing. While this somewhat daunting situation is being sorted out by the more academically inclined, empirical frontal approaches are being enthusiastically followed in many centres. One major strategy is to reduce the tumour load by surgery, irradiation or chemotherapy and then to immunize with irradiated tumour cells in conjunction with an adjuvant such as B.C.G. or killed *Corynebacterium parvum*. Another attack based on the not unreasonable belief that certain forms of cancer, (e.g. leukaemia) are caused by oncogenic viruses, envisages attempts to isolate the virus and prepare a suitable vaccine from it. Efforts in this direction involving large scale vaccination of poultry against Marek's disease with the relevant DNA virus look encouraging. In the end it may turn out that almost any attempt to increase the immune response of the host to his tumour (either by heightening his own responsive-ness with general adjuvants, transfer factor etc. or by increasing the antigenicity of the tumour through modification or coupl-ing to a carrier) will prove beneficial but in the meantime the gloomy prognostication that we may generate harmful blocking factors should not be disregarded. There is also growing suspicion that activation of non-specific cytotoxic activity of macrophages may contribute to the therapeutic response of some tumours to adjuvants.

IMMUNODIAGNOSIS

Analysis of blood for the oncofoetal antigens α-foetoprotein in hepatoma and carcinoembryonic antigen in tumours of the colon has provided valuable diagnostic information but en-thusiasm has been slightly curtailed by the knowledge that there is a high incidence of so-called 'false positives'. Caspary & Field have developed a test which depends on the observation that lymphocytes from cancer patients when mixed with a basic protein commonly found in tumours, will release a factor which slows the electrophoretic mobility of added macrophages. The technique of cytopherometry which must be employed is fiddly and there has been some ambivalence in coming to terms with what could potentially become a powerful diagnostic tool. Another line of research places its faith in the idea that a variety of long term tumour cell lines could provide a comprehensive test kit to monitor the lymphocytes from apparently normal people for heightened reactivity to tumour antigens *in vitro*.

Other biological properties of transplantation antigens

It is tempting to speculate that the major transplantation antigens subserve a primitive recognition function. Cells from a given tissue have some mechanism by which they recognize each other. For example, dispersed kidney cells in culture together with hepatocytes preferentially reaggregate with each other. This process of recognition and adherence might be mediated through tissue-specific surface antigens which could conceivably be related to or part of the molecules bearing the major transplantation antigens.

The phenomenon of *allogeneic inhibition* is cited as evidence that histocompatibility antigens may initiate intercellular reactions independently of conventionally recognized immunological mechanisms and could thereby act to destroy tumour cells or at least to limit their growth rate. For example, despite the fact that F_1 hybrids (AB) will not react against parental strain cells (A or B) in the usual skin graft or graft vs. host situations, tumour cells grow better in syngeneic hosts than in semi-syngeneic F_1 hybrids. Furthermore, F_1 lymphocytes mixed with phytohaemagglutin are activated to prevent growth of monolayer cultures of parental strain fibroblasts whereas syngeneic parental strain lymphocytes are not. Before rejecting a conventional immunological explanation two possibilities have to be excluded: (i) a recessive gene in the parental strain coding for a histocompatibility antigen and (ii) creation of a new antigenic specificity on the cell surface by the juxtaposition of two A antigens in the parent as compared with A and B in the F_1 hybrid. Another type of cellular interaction, T-B co-operation, is strongly influenced by the nature of the

208

histocompatibility antigens in so far as the phenomenon does not occur when the co-operating cells differ at the major loci.

In the mouse the H-2 region of the chromosome is bound up with recognition in the sense that the subregions of the immune response genes Ir-1A and Ir-1B lie between the two major H-2 loci (figure 8.4). Whether the H-2 gene contributes a peptide to the recognition unit is not known. It is of interest that β_2-microglobulin which is found in the urine in certain conditions and shows considerable homology with the constant region domains of immunoglobulin, appears to represent a part of the HL-A molecule.

An impressive body of data is accumulating which links specific HL-A antigens with particular disease states in the human. Of these perhaps the most notable is the extraordinarily high frequency of HL-A27 in patients with ankylosing spondylitis and other conditions involving sacro-ileitis. Other examples are the association of HL-A1 and HL-A8 with coeliac disease and active chronic hepatitis and of HL-A13 and HL-A17 with psoriasis. There are many more. Because of linkage disequilibrium (a state where closely linked genes on a chromosome tend to remain associated rather than undergo genetic drift) which is often a feature of this region of the chromosome, the associations seen may be even more directly linked with genes other than HL-A itself, e.g. Ir genes or those controlling androgen levels or others not yet identified.

Experiments with synchronized lymphoid tumour cell populations have revealed cyclical changes in the surface density of histocompatibility antigens, which falls to minimum values during the DNA synthetic phase of the mitotic cycle.

This region of the chromosome is characterized by multiple alleles and it may be that polymorphism in these antigens helps to guard a species against the danger that a pathogenic organism may evolve antigens closely similar to those of the host and so avoid provoking an immune reaction.

Immunological relationship of mother and foetus

Because the foetus derives transplantation antigens from the father as well as the mother, it represents a potential graft. Intrigued by this notion, Lewis Thomas was moved to suggest that transplantation rejection of the foetus might initiate parturition although it would be difficult to account for the normal birth of female offspring to pure strain mating pairs (foetus and mother have identical histocompatibility antigens) without further postulating a placenta-specific surface antigen.

Nonetheless in the human haemochorial placenta, maternal blood with immunocompetent lymphocytes does circulate in contact with the foetal trophoblast and we have to explain how the foetus avoids allograft rejection. Prior sensitization with a skin graft fails to affect a pregnancy, suggesting that the trophoblast cells may be immunologically privileged. Although these cells bear paternal antigens it may be that their surface density is relatively low. This might result in the trophoblast being only weakly antigenic or perhaps might lead to the formation of enhancing factors as suggested by the work of Hellström. Furthermore, the cells possess an outer layer of mucopolysaccharide rich in sialic acid, which although not complete, could act as a barrier to attack by sensitized lymphocytes. Immunological processes do somehow affect the placenta in that mothers tolerant to paternal antigens have smaller placentae than mothers previously sensitized to these antigens.

The production of haemolytic disease of the newborn and of possible g.v.h. reactions in the foetus by placental transfer of Rh antibodies in the one case and maternal lymphocytes in the other, have already been discussed.

Further reading

Batchelor J.R. & Brent L. (1971) Histocompatibility in transplantation immunity. In Borek F. (ed) *Immunogenicity*. North Holland, Amsterdam.

Billingham R. & Silvers W. (1971) *The Immunobiology of Transplantation*. Foundations of Immunology Series, Prentice-Hall, N. Jersey.

Brent L. (1972) Tolerance and enhancement in organ transplantation. *Transpl. Proc.*, **4**, 363.

Burnet F.M. (1970) Relationship of diversity in histocompatibility antigens to immunological surveillance mechanisms for control of cancer. *Nature*, **226**, 123.

Dausset J. & Hors J. (1973) Statistics of 416 consecutive kidney transplants in the France-Transplant organization. *Transpl. Proc.*, **5**, 223.

Lance E.M., Medawar P.B. & Taub R.N. (1973) Antilymphocyte serum. *Adv. in Immunology*, **17**, 2.

Landy M. & Smith R.T. (eds) (1971) *Immunological Surveillance*. Brook Lodge Symposium, Academic Press, London.

Mitchison N.A. (1973) Tumour-immunology. In Roitt I. (ed) *Essays in Fundamental Immunology 1*, page 44. Blackwell Scientific Publications, Oxford

Russell P.S. & Winn H.J. (1970) Transplantation: a review. *N. Eng. J. Med.*, **282**, 786, 848 and 896.

Skinner M.D. & Schwartz R.S. (1972) Immunosuppressive Therapy. *N. Eng. J. Med.*, **287**, 221 and 281

(1973) Genetic and biological aspects of histocompatibility antigens. *Transpl. Rev. No. 16.*

9   Autoimmunity

There are in the body appropriate mechanisms to prevent the recognition of 'self' components as antigens by the lymphoid system but, as with all machinery, there is always a chance that these mechanisms might break down, and the older the individual, the greater the chance of a breakdown. When this happens *autoantibodies* (i.e. antibodies capable of reacting with 'self' components) are produced. Grabar is of the opinion that auto-antibodies have a biological function to act as 'transporting' agents for cellular breakdown products thereby aiding their disposal. While antibodies can act in this way, we are here concerned more with autoimmune phenomena which appear in relation to certain defined human diseases. Ideally we wish to apply the term 'autoimmune disease' to those cases where it can be shown that the autoimmune process contributes to the pathogenesis of the disease rather than situations where apparently harmless autoantibodies are formed following tissue damage, e.g. heart antibodies appearing after a myocardial infarction. Yet the role of autoimmunity in many disorders is still not clearly defined, and it is as a matter of convenience that we will refer to all maladies firmly associated with autoantibody formation as 'autoimmune diseases', except where it can be shown that the immunological phenomena are purely secondary findings.

The spectrum of autoimmune diseases

These disorders may be looked upon as forming a spectrum. At one end we have '*organ-specific diseases*' with organ-specific autoantibodies. Hashimoto's disease of the thyroid is an example: there is a specific lesion in the thyroid involving infiltration by mononuclear cells (lymphocytes, histiocytes and plasma cells), destruction of follicular cells and germinal centre formation, accompanied by the production of circulating antibodies with absolute specificity for certain thyroid constituents (Roitt & Doniach).

Moving towards the centre of the spectrum are those disorders where the lesion tends to be localized to a single organ but the antibodies are non-organ specific. A typical example would be primary biliary cirrhosis where the small bile ductule is the main target of inflammatory cell infiltration but the serum antibodies present—mainly mitochondrial—are not liver specific.

At the other end of the spectrum are the '*non-organ specific diseases*' exemplified by systemic lupus erythematosus (SLE) where both lesions and autoantibodies are not confined to any one organ. Pathological changes are widespread and are primarily lesions of connective tissue with fibrinoid necrosis. They are seen in the skin (the 'lupus' butterfly rash on the face is characteristic), kidney glomeruli, joints, serous membranes and blood vessels. In addition the formed elements of the blood are often affected. A bizarre collection of autoantibodies are found some of which react with the DNA and other nuclear constituents of all cells in the body.

An attempt to fit the major diseases considered to be associated with autoimmunity into this spectrum is shown in table 9.1.

TABLE 9.1. Spectrum of autoimmune diseases

Organ specific ←				→ Non-organ specific
Hashimoto's thyroiditis	Goodpasture's syndrome	Myasthenia gravis	Primary biliary cirrhosis	Systemic lupus erythematosus
Primary myxoedema	Pemphigus vulgaris	Autoimmune haemolytic anaemia	Active chronic hepatitis (some cases)	(SLE) Discoid LE
Thyrotoxicosis	Pemphigoid	Idiopathic thrombocytopenic	Cryptogenic	Dermatomyositis Scleroderma
Pernicious anaemia	Sympathetic ophthalmia	purpura	cirrhosis (some	Rheumatoid
Autoimmune atrophic gastritis	Phacogenic uveitis	Idiopathic leucopenia	cases)	arthritis
Addison's disease			Ulcerative colitis	
Premature menopause (few cases)			Sjögren's syndrome	
Male infertility (few cases)	(?? Multiple sclerosis ??)			

Autoantibodies in human disease

At this stage in the discussion it may be of value to have a more precise account of the major autoantibodies detected in the different diseases to provide a framework for reference. Table 9.2 documents a list of these antibodies and the methods employed in their detection. The notes following the table amplify specific points while some of the tests are illustrated in figures 9.1–9.4.

TABLE 9.2. Autoantibodies in human disease
(IFT = Immunofluorescent test; CFT = complement fixation test)

Disease	Antigen	Detection of antibody
Hashimoto's thyroiditis ⎱ Primary myxoedema ⎰	Thyroglobulin	Precipitins; passive haemaggln. IFT on fixed thyroid
	2nd Colloid Ag (CA2)	IFT on fixed thyroid
	Cytoplasmic microsomes	IFT on unfixed thyroid; CFT with thyroid microsomes
	Cell surface	IFT on viable thyroid cells; C′-mediated cytotoxicity
Thyrotoxicosis	Probably cell surface	Bioassay—stimulation of mouse thyroid *in vivo*
Pernicious anaemia[1]	Intrinsic factor	Neutralization; blocking combination with vit-B_{12}; binding to Int.Fact-B_{12} by copptn.
	Parietal cell microsomes	IFT on unfixed gastric mucosa; CFT with mucosal homogenate
Addison's disease	Cytoplasm adrenal cells	IFT on unfixed adrenal cortex; CFT
Premature onset of menopause[2]	Cytoplasm steroid producing cells	IFT on adrenal and interstitial cells of ovary and testis
Male infertility (some)[3]	Spermatozoa	Sperm agglutination in ejaculate
(Multiple Sclerosis)	Brain	Cytotoxic effects on cerebellar cultures by serum and lymphocytes (? secondary to disease)
Goodpasture's syndrome	Glomerular and lung basement membrane	Linear staining by IFT of kidney biopsy with fluorescent anti-IgG
Pemphigus vulgaris	Desmosomes between prickle cells in epidermis	IFT on skin
Pemphigoid	Basement membrane	IFT on skin
Phacogenic uveitis	Lens	Passive haemagglutination
Sympathetic ophthalmia	Uvea	(Delayed skin reaction to uveal extract)
Myasthenia gravis	Skeletal and heart muscle; thymus myoid cells	IFT on skeletal muscle
Autoimmune haemolytic anaemia[4]	Erythrocytes	Coombs' antiglobulin test
Idiopathic thrombocytopenic purpura	Platelets	Shortened platelet survival *in vivo*
Primary biliary cirrhosis	Mitochondria (mainly)	IFT on mitochondria rich cells (e.g. distal tubules of kidney); CFT kidney

Table 9.2 (*contd.*)

Disease	Antigen	Detection of antibody
Active chronic hepatitis	Smooth muscle, nuclei (mainly)	IFT (e.g. on gastric mucosa)
Ulcerative colitis	Colon 'lipopoly-saccharide'	IFT; passive haemaggln. (cytotoxic action of lymphocytes on colon cells)
Sjögren's syndrome[5]	Ducts, mitochondria, nuclei, thyroid, IgG	IFT; antiglobulin tests
Rheumatoid arthritis[6]	IgG	Antiglobulin tests: latex aggln. and sheep red cell aggln. test (SCAT)
	? microorganisms	
Discoid lupus erythematosus ⎫	Nuclear	IFT
Dermatomyositis ⎬	IgG	Antiglobulin tests
Scleroderma[7] ⎭		
Systemic lupus erythematosus	DNA	Pptn.; CFT; IFT; Farr
	Nucleoprotein	IFT; latex aggln. L.E. cells[8]
	Cytoplasmic sol.Ag	'Non-organ sp.CFT'
	Array of other Ag incl. formed elements of blood, clotting factors, altered IgG and Wasserman antigen	'Biological false positive' CFT

Notes:

1. Two major types of antibody to intrinsic factor are detected, viz. blocking and binding (figure 9.1). Binding antibody combines with preformed Int.Fact.—radio-active B_{12}($^xB_{12}$) complex which can then be precipitated at 50 per cent ammonium sulphate (cf. Farr test—salt copptn., p. 106) and the radioactivity in the precipitate counted. Blocking antibody prevents binding of $^xB_{12}$ to Int.Fact. and the uncombined $^xB_{12}$ can then be adsorbed on charcoal and counted.

2. Antibodies occur in the minority of patients with associated Addison's disease.

3. Only small percentage show agglutinins. Spermatozoa may be agglutinated head to head, tail to tail or joined through their mid-piece. Seen also in small percentage of infertile women.

4. The Coombs' test involves the demonstration of bound antibody on the washed red cell by agglutination with an antiglobulin. Erythrocyte autoantibodies, which bind well over the temperature range $0-37°C$ ('warm' Ab), are mostly IgG; approximately 60 per cent of cases are primary, the remainder being associated with other auto-immune disorders, e.g. SLE, ulcerative colitis. 'Cold' Ab, which react best over the range $0-20°C$, are mostly IgM and red cells coated with this Ab can often be agglutin-ated by anti-complement sera; approximately half are primary, the others being associated with *Mycoplasma pneumoniae* infection or generalized neoplastic disease of the lymphoreticular tissues.

5. Antibodies specifically reacting with the epithelium of salivary gland excretory ducts are demonstrable by immunofluorescence in up to half the cases.

6. The main antiglobulin factors react with the Fc portion of IgG which is usually adsorbed onto latex particles (human IgG) or present in an antigen–antibody complex (sheep red cells coated with subagglutinating dose of rabbit antibody).

7. In scleroderma (progressive systemic sclerosis) antinucleolar antibodies are frequently found.

8. When blood from an SLE patient is incubated at $37°C$, some white cells are damaged and allow the entry of antibodies. Certain of the antibodies combining with the nuclear surface bind complement and attract polymorphs which strip away the cytoplasm and engulf the nucleus. The polymorph containing the engulfed homogenized nucleus is called an LE-cell (figure 9.4).

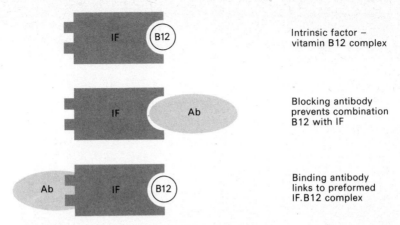

IF   B12
Intrinsic factor –
vitamin B12 complex

IF   Ab
Blocking antibody
prevents combination
B12 with IF

Ab   IF   B12
Binding antibody
links to preformed
IF.B12 complex

FIGURE 9.1. Intrinsic factor autoantibodies: sites of determinants for binding and blocking.

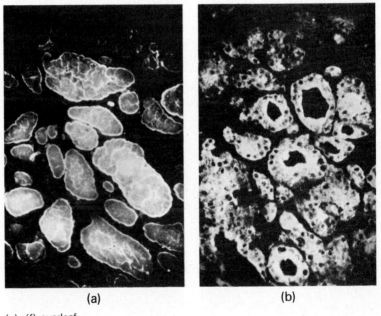

(a)   (b)

(c)–(f) overleaf

FIGURE 9.2. Autoantibodies demonstrable by immunofluorescent test:
(a) thyroglobulin antibodies reacting with colloid of fixed thyroid section;
(b) thyroid microsomal antibodies staining cytoplasm of acinar cells;
(c) serum of patient with Addison's disease staining cytoplasm of adrenal
cells; (d) striated muscle antibodies in serum of patient with myasthenia
gravis reacting with 'myoid' cell in human thymus; (e) fluorescence of
distal tubular cells of the kidney after reaction with mitochondrial autoantibodies; (f) diffuse nuclear staining obtained with nucleoprotein
antibodies on a thyroid section. ((d) kindly provided by Dr. T.E.W.
Feltkamp, the others by courtesy of Dr. D. Doniach.)

215

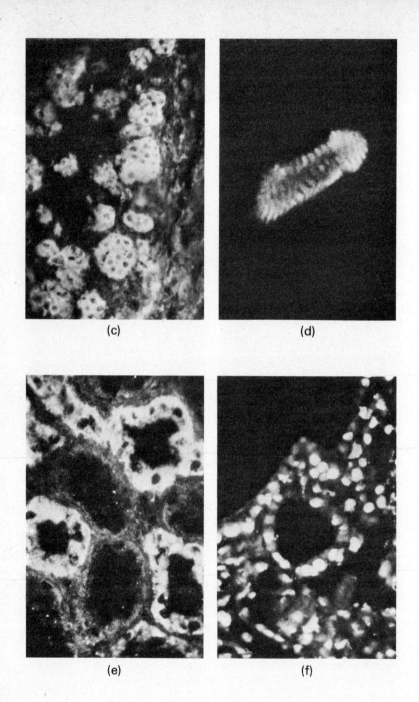

(c)

(d)

(e)

(f)

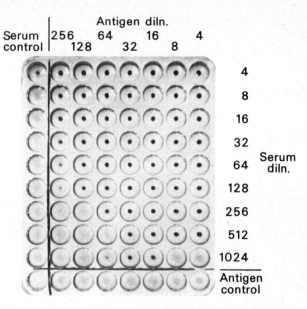

FIGURE 9.3. Complement fixation test showing reaction of antibodies from Hashimoto patient with thyroid homogenate. Serial dilutions of antigen and antiserum have been used in a checkerboard titration. A button of unlysed indicator cells at the bottom of a cup is indicative of complement fixation (cf. p. 119). The serum gives positive fixation at a dilution of 1 : 1,024 with antigen dilutions of 1 : 16 or 1 : 32.

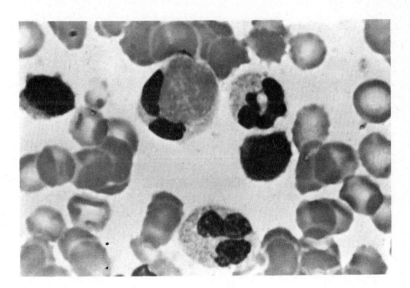

FIGURE 9.4. LE-cell in preparation from peripheral blood of SLE patient. The homogeneous nucleus lies within the polymorph which engulfed it by phagocytosis. Two normal polymorphs and two small lymphocytes are also present. (Photographed from material kindly provided by Prof. J.W. Stewart.)

Overlap of autoimmune disorders

There is a tendency for more than one autoimmune disorder to occur in the same individual and when this happens the association is often between diseases within the same region of the autoimmune spectrum (cf. table 9.1). Thus patients with auto-immune thyroiditis (Hashimoto's disease or primary myx-oedema) have a much higher incidence of pernicious anaemia than would be expected in a random population matched for age and sex (10 per cent as against 0·2 per cent). Conversely both thyroiditis and thyrotoxicosis are diagnosed in pernicious anaemia patients with an unexpectedly high frequency. Other associations are seen with Addison's disease and autoimmune thyroid disease and in the rare cases of juveniles with pernicious anaemia and polyendocrinopathy which includes Addison's disease, hypoparathyroidism and thyroiditis.

There is an even greater overlap in serological findings. Thirty per cent of patients with autoimmune thyroid disease have con-comitant parietal cell antibodies in their serum. Conversely, thyroid antibodies have been demonstrated in up to 50 per cent of pernicious anaemia patients. It should be stressed that these are not cross-reacting antibodies. The thyroid specific anti-bodies will not react with stomach and *vice versa*. When a serum reacts with both organs it means that two populations of antibodies are present, one with specificity for thyroid and the other for stomach.

TABLE 9.3. Organ-specific and non-organ-specific serological interrelationships in human disease

Disease	% Positive reactions for antibodies to:				
	Thyroid*	Stomach*·	Nuclei*	Non-organ-specific antigen**	IgG†
Hashimoto's thyroiditis	99·9	32	8	5	2
Pernicious anaemia	55	89	11	7	
Sjögren's syndrome	45	14	56	19	75
Rheumatoid arthritis	11	16	50	10	75
S.L.E.	2	2	99	66	35
Controls‡	0–15	0–16	0–19	0–10	2–5

* Immunofluorescence test   ** CFT with kidney   † Rheumatoid factor classical tests
‡ Incidence increases with age and females > males

At the non-organic-specific end of the spectrum, SLE is clinically associated with rheumatoid arthritis and several other diseases which are themselves uncommon: haemolytic anaemia, idiopathic leucopenia and thrombocytopenic purpura, dermatomyositis and Sjögren's syndrome. Antinuclear antibodies, non-organ-specific complement fixation reactions, and anti-globulin (rheumatoid) factors are a general feature of these disorders.

Sjögren's syndrome occupies an interesting position (table 9.3); aside from the clinical and serological features associated with non-organ-specific disease mentioned above, characteristics of an organ-specific disorder are evident. Antibodies reacting with salivary ducts are demonstrable and there is an abnormally high incidence of thyroid autoantibodies; histologically the affected lacrimal and salivary glands reveal changes of a similar nature to those seen in Hashimoto's disease, namely a replacement of the glandular elements by patchy lymphocytic and plasma cell granulomatous tissue. Associations between diseases at the two ends of the spectrum have been reported, but they are rare as might be predicted from the serological data (table 9.3).

There is still no entirely satisfactory explanation to account for the rare tendency to develop hypogammaglobulinaemia and the increased incidence of certain cancers occurring in auto-immune disease. Patients with organ specific disorders are slightly more prone to develop cancer in the affected organ whereas generalized lymphoreticular neoplasia shows up with uncommon frequency in non-organ-specific disease.

Genetic factors in autoimmune disease

Autoimmune phenomena tend to aggregate in certain families. For example, the first degree relatives (sibs, parents and children) of patients with Hashimoto's disease show a high incidence of thyroid autoantibodies and of overt and subclinical thyroiditis. Parallel studies have disclosed similar relationships in the families of pernicious anaemia patients in that gastric parietal cell antibodies are prevalent in the relatives who are wont to develop achlorhydria and atrophic gastritis. A somewhat unusual family is depicted in figure 9.5 which illustrates these features and reminds us of the thyroid–stomach link. Familial aggregation of mitochondrial antibodies has been observed, albeit to a lesser extent, in primary biliary cirrhosis. Turning to SLE, disturbances of immunoglobulin synthesis

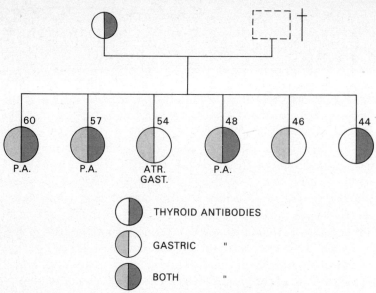

FIGURE 9.5. Familial aggregation of gastric autoimmunity. Six female siblings with their respective ages and autoantibodies are shown. Three had pernicious anaemia (PA) and another atrophic gastritis (Atr.gast.). The mother had myxoedema. (Courtesy Dr. D. Doniach).

and a susceptibility to develop 'connective tissue diseases' have been reported but there are some conflicting accounts still not resolved.

These familial relationships could be ascribed to environmental factors such as an infective micro-organism, but there is evidence that a genetic component must be given some consideration. In the first place, when thyrotoxicosis occurs in twins there is a greater concordance rate (i.e. both twins affected) in identical than in non-identical twins. Secondly, thyroid autoantibodies are more prevalent in individuals with ovarian dysgenesis having X-chromosome aberrations such as XO and particularly the isochromosome X abnormality. Furthermore, pure strain animals have been bred which spontaneously develop autoimmune disease. There is an obese line of chickens with autoimmune thyroiditis and the New Zealand Black (NZB) mouse with autoimmune haemolytic anaemia. The hybrid of NZB with another strain the New Zealand White (BxW hybrid) actually develops LE-cells, antinuclear antibodies and a fatal immune complex induced glomerulonephritis. Suitable intercross and backcross breeding of these creatures has established that a *minimum* of three genes determines the expression of autoimmunity and that the production of both red cell and nuclear antibodies may be under separate genetic control.

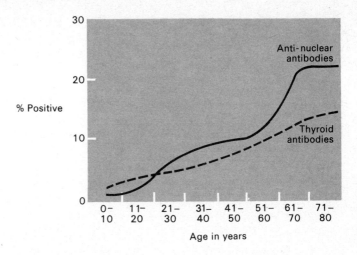

FIGURE 9.6. Incidence of autoantibodies in the general population. A serum was considered positive for thyroid antibodies if it reacted at a dilution of 1/10 in the tanned red cell test or neat in the immunofluorescent test and positive for antinuclear antibodies if it reacted at a dilution of 1/4 by immunofluorescence.

Autoantibodies are demonstrable in comparatively low titre in the general population and the incidence of positive results increases steadily with age (figure 9.6) up to around 60–70 years. In the case of the thyroid and stomach at least, biopsy has indicated that the presence of antibody is almost invariably associated with minor thyroiditis or gastritis lesions (as the case may be), and it is of interest that post mortem examination has identified 10 per cent of middle-aged women with significant degrees of lymphadenoid change in the thyroid similar in essence to that characteristic of Hashimoto's disease. The point may also be made here that in general autoantibodies and autoimmune diseases are found more frequently in women than in men.

Aetiology of autoimmune response

How do autoantibodies arise? Our earliest view, with respect to organ specific antibodies at least, was that the antigens were sequestered within the organ and through lack of contact with the lymphoreticular system failed to establish immunological tolerance. Any mishap which caused a release of the antigen would then provide an opportunity for autoantibody formation.

For a few body constituents this holds true and in the case of sperm and heart for example, release of certain components directly into the circulation can provoke autoantibodies. But in general, the experience has been that injection of *unmodified* extracts of those tissues concerned in the organ-specific auto-immune disorders does not elicit antibody formation. Indeed detailed investigation of the thyroid autoantigen, thyroglobulin, has disclosed that it is not completely sequestered within the gland but gains access to the extracellular fluid around the follicles and leaves via the thyroid lymphatics (figure 9.7) reaching the serum in normal human subjects at concentrations of approximately 0·01–0·05 μg/ml.

Concentrations of this order produce 'low zone tolerance' in mice probably by affecting the T-lymphocytes. Extrapolating to man, we are presumably dealing with a situation in which T-cells are tolerant to thyroglobulin and B-cells are not. Indeed a small proportion of the B-cells in normal individuals bind human thyroglobulin; and this may be true for many different body constituents. In terms of autoantibody production there are only four antigenic determinants on human thyroglobulin

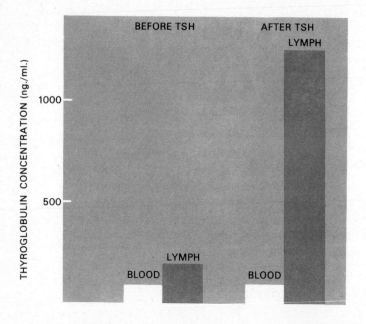

FIGURE 9.7. Thyroglobulin in the cervical lymph draining the thyroid in the rat. The concentration of thyroglobulin is increased after injection of pituitary thyroid stimulating hormone (TSH) suggesting that the release from thyroid follicles is linked to the physiological activity of the acinar cells (from Daniel P.N., Pratt O.E., Roitt I.M. & Torrigiani G., *Quart.J.exp.Physiol.* 1967, **52**, 184).

(mol. wt. 650,000) and these may behave merely as haptenic groups in the sense that the non-tolerant B-cells can only be stimulated by these groups through T-cell co-operation. Because the T-cells are tolerant to thyroglobulin, the B-lymphocytes will not normally be activated.

There are a number of ways in which this situation might be bypassed:

(i) *Modification of the molecule*

One mechanism would be through the presentation of these potentially autoantigenic determinants on a new carrier (figure 9.8) (cf. Weigle's work on termination of tolerance; chapter 3). This could arise through some modifications to the molecule, for example, by an abnormality in lysosomal break-down yielding a split product exposing some new groupings. Experimentally it has been found that large proteolytic frag-ments of thyroglobulin are autoantigenic when injected alone but no evidence for such a mechanism has yet been uncovered in man; where antibodies to a split product such as the $F(ab')_2$ fragment of IgG have been detected, they have not reacted with the whole molecule.

Incorporation into Freund's complete adjuvant frequently endows these molecules with autoantigenic properties and as we shall see later this enables us to induce many autoallergic diseases in laboratory animals. It is conceivable that the physical constraints on the proteins at the water–oil interface of the emulsion provide the required alteration in configuration of the 'carrier portions' of the molecules.

Modification can also be achieved through combination with a drug. The autoimmune haemolytic anaemia associated with administration of α-methyl dopa might be attributable to modi-fication of the red-cell surface in such a way as to provide a carrier for stimulating B-cells which recognize the Rhesus *e* antigen. This is normally regarded as a 'weak' antigen and would be less likely to induce B-cell tolerance than the 'stronger' antigens present on the erythrocyte.

(ii) *Cross-reactions*

Many examples are known in which potential autoantigenic determinants are present on an exogenous cross-reacting anti-gen and can provoke autoantibody formation, again presumably by the mechanism depicted in figure 9.8. Post rabies vaccine encephalitis is thought to result from an autoimmune reaction

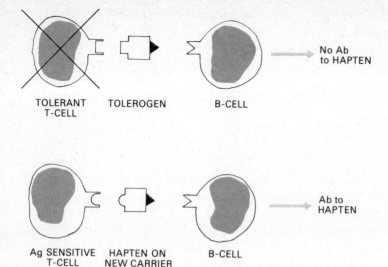

No Ab
to HAPTEN

TOLERANT   TOLEROGEN   B-CELL
T-CELL

Ab to
HAPTEN

Ag SENSITIVE   HAPTEN ON   B-CELL
T-CELL   NEW CARRIER

FIGURE 9.8. Termination of unresponsiveness to hapten (▶) induced by
hapten-protein conjugate, by hapten on new carrier (Weigle/Allison model). If
autologous thyroglobulin is considered as a tolerogen inducing unresponsiveness in T-cells but leaving B-cells capable of reacting with small
determinants on the molecule (equivalent to hapten because these will not
be antigenic if T-cell co-operation is required), then a different molecule
bearing these determinants will provoke autoantibody production by
providing a new carrier which can be recognized as foreign by other
T-cells.

to brain initiated by heterologous brain tissue in the vaccine (cf.
experimental allergic encephalomyelitis below). Some micro-
organisms carry determinants which cross-react with the
human and this may prove to be an important way of inducing
autoimmunity. In rheumatic fever antibodies produced to the
streptococcus also react with heart, and colon antibodies present
in ulcerative colitis have been found to cross-react with
Escherichia coli 014.

(iii) *Other effects of micro-organisms*

Non-cross-reacting microbes could still subserve a carrier
function by providing immunogenic molecules closely attached
to potential autoantigens. Perhaps *Mycoplasma pneumoniae*
modifies the erythrocyte in this way and leads to production of
cold agglutinins. The nucleic acid in a DNA virus might
become antigenic by virtue of its association with immunogenic
viral proteins and virally infected cells sometimes carry new
antigens on their surface.

Micro-organisms often act as adjuvants through their possession of constituents such as bacterial glycolipids and endo-toxins which may act by providing the second (non-specific) inductive signal for B-cell stimulation (cf. figure 3.9d), so bypassing the need for T-cell help. The possibility that lymphoid cells become abnormally modified by viral infection is discussed below.

(iv) *Abnormal lymphoid system*

If the mechanism for tolerance induction were to fail, then autoreactive lymphocytes (described as 'forbidden clones' by Burnet) would be generated. This might happen through somatic mutation or infection of the lymphoid system by a virus.

It is worthy of note that cell lines (θ+ve, Ig−ve i.e. probably T-cell) established from NZB mice shed tremendous amounts of a C type oncornavirus which appears to be leukaemogenic and capable of inducing early antinuclear antibodies and glomerulonephritis on transfer to Balb/c × NZB F1 hybrids. The replication of such an RNA virus through the reverse transcriptase pathway seems to be reflected in the finding of autoantibodies with specificity for single and double stranded RNA and DNA, and for an RNA-DNA hybrid. It should soon be possible to decide whether this virus is capable of disturbing the orderly function of the immune system and there is no doubt that the links between autoimmune disease, immunoglobin abnormalities and cancer would be more readily comprehensible were such an underlying disturbance to be recognized.

Regulation of the immune response by 'suppressor' T-cells was discussed in chapter 3 and there are many pointers to defective T-lymphocyte function in autoimmune states—certainly in the spontaneous animal models. Neonatal thymectomy exacerbates the thyroiditis in obese chickens and the autoimmune haemolytic anaemia and glomerulonephritis of NZB mice. The onset of disease in these mice can be largely prevented by repeated injections of thymocytes from young unaffected animals and conversely spleen cells transferred from diseased to young NZB mice only continue to synthesize auto-antibodies for a short time unless the recipients are first immunosuppressed. In other words, the young T-cells appear to exert a controlling influence on the autoantibody-producing B-cells. The increased difficulty in establishing T-cell tolerance to an exogenous antigen and the sharp fall in thymus hormone concentration in the blood as these mice become diseased provide yet further examples of thymus dysfunction.

Pathogenic mechanisms in autoimmune disease

We have mentioned that despite certain exceptions as, for instance, myocardial infarction or damage to the testis, traumatic release of organ constituents does not in general elicit antibody formation. Destruction of thyroid tissue by therapeutic doses of radio-iodine does not initiate thyroid autoimmunity nor does damage to the liver in alcoholic cirrhosis result in the synthesis of mitochondrial antibodies, to give but two examples. We should now look at the evidence which bears directly on the issue of whether autoimmunity, however it arises, plays a *primary* pathogenic role in the production of tissue lesions in the group of diseases labelled as 'autoimmune'.

EFFECTS OF HUMORAL ANTIBODY

Blood

The erythrocyte antibodies play a role in the destruction of red cells in autoimmune haemolytic anaemia. Normal red cells coated with autoantibody eluted from Coombs' positive erythrocytes have a shortened half life after reinjection into the normal subject. Normal red cells also have a shortened survival when infused into patients with haemolytic anaemia, but only if they possess the antigens against which the patient's autoantibodies are directed showing that the destructive process must be linked to the autoimmune response. Platelet antibodies are apparently responsible for idiopathic thrombocytopenic purpura (ITP). IgG from a patient's serum when given to a normal individual causes a depression of platelet counts and the active principle can be absorbed out with platelets. The transient neonatal thrombocytopenia which may be seen in infants of mothers with ITP is explicable in terms of transplacental passage of IgG antibodies to the child.

Some children with immunodeficiency associated with very low white cell counts have a serum lymphocytotoxic factor which requires complement for its activity. Lymphopenia occurring in patients with SLE and rheumatoid arthritis may also be a direct result of antibody since non-agglutinating antibodies coating the white cells have been reported.

Thyroid

Cytotoxic antibodies. The serum of patients with Hashimoto's disease is cytotoxic for human thyroid cells growing in mono-

226

layer culture after dispersal by trypsin. This is a typical complement-mediated antibody reaction directed against cell surface antigens but it is still difficult to assess the extent to which this can operate *in vivo*. In the first place, simple fragments of thyroid gland grow out well in medium containing cytotoxic antibody and complement which raises the possibility that trypsin-treatment to obtain monolayers may either expose surface determinants that are normally protected or make the cells more fragile and susceptible to cytotoxic attack. Secondly, there is no evidence that infants born to Hashimoto mothers have defective thyroid function despite the presence of the antibody in their serum.

Long-acting thyroid stimulator. Under certain circumstances antibodies to the surface of a cell may stimulate rather than destroy (cf. type V sensitivity; chapter 6). This would seem to be the case in thyrotoxicosis (Graves' or Basedow's disease). There has long been indirect evidence suggesting a link between autoimmune processes and this disease: thyroid antibodies are detectable in up to 85 per cent of thyrotoxic patients and histologically the majority of the glands removed at operation show varying degrees of thyroiditis in addition to the characteristic acinar cell hyperplasia (figure 9.9); thyrotoxicosis is found with undue frequency in the families of Hashimoto patients; there is an association with gastric auto-

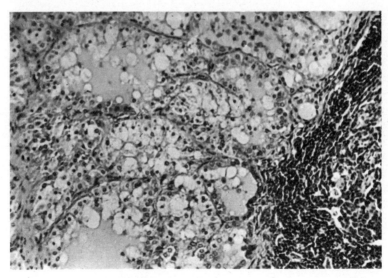

FIGURE 9.9. Lymphoid follicle adjacent to hyperactive thyroid cells representing histological features of thyroiditis and Graves' disease in gland taken from patient with thyrotoxicosis.

immunity in that 30 per cent have gastric antibodies and up to 10 per cent pernicious anaemia. The direct link came with the discovery by Adams and Purves of thyroid stimulating activity in the serum of thyrotoxic patients. Using a new bioassay they showed that the serum caused a stimulation of the thyroid gland of the recipient animal which was considerably prolonged relative to the time course of action of the physiological thyroid stimulating hormone (TSH) from the pituitary (figure 9.10). This long-acting thyroid stimulator (LATS) has all the attributes of a thyroid-specific antibody:

(a) Activity is recovered in the IgG fraction.

(b) Fab and $F(ab')_2$ fragments are stimulatory but not the Fc.

(c) Isolated heavy and light chains are virtually inactive but significant LATS activity is recovered on recombination.

(d) Activity can be absorbed out by homogenates of thyroid but not other organs, and can be eluted afterwards from the homogenate by acid treatment which would be expected to dissociate antibody in combination with its antigen.

(e) LATS crosses the placenta and produces neonatal hyperthyroidism which resolves after a few weeks as the maternal IgG is catabolized.

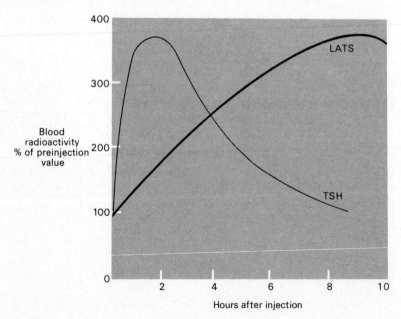

FIGURE 9.10. Bioassay of long-acting thyroid stimulator (LATS). The release of ^{131}I from the prelabelled thyroid of the recipient animal is prolonged relative to the action of TSH.

228

LATS seems to act on the thyroid in the same manner as TSH, perhaps by stimulating identical receptors (cf. figure 6.14). Both operate through the adenyl cyclase system as indicated by the potentiating effect of theophylline, and both produce very similar changes in ultrastructural morphology in the thyroid cell. Because LATS acts independently of the pituitary–thyroid axis, iodine uptake by the gland is unaffected by administration of thyroxine or tri-iodothyronine, whereas normally this would cause feedback inhibition and suppression of uptake (figure 9.11); this forms the basis of an important diagnostic test for thyrotoxicosis.

A pathogenetic role for LATS has been questioned on the grounds that the sera from at least 20% of active thyrotoxic patients do not give positive assays for this factor in mice (the normal test animal) even when IgG concentrates are tested. However, it now appears that IgG from these negative sera can stimulate colloid droplet formation in cultured slices of *human* thyroid and furthermore can act as an 'LATS' protector' in the sense that it can coat human thyroid microsomes and so prevent them from neutralizing a positive LATS serum. The implication is that the LATS-negative sera contain a stimulating anti-human thyroid antibody which fails to cross-react with the gland of the assay animal.

Intrinsic factor

Autoantibodies to this product of gastric mucosal secretion were first demonstrated in pernicious anaemia patients by oral

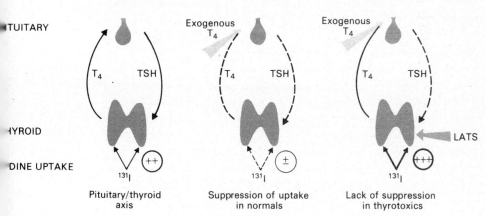

FIGURE 9.11. Suppression test in thyrotoxicosis. Administration of thyroxine (T_4) in normals inhibits pituitary secretion of TSH and suppresses iodine uptake. TSH output is diminished in thyrotoxicosis even without administration of thyroxine because LATS constantly stimulates the thyroid.

229

administration of intrinsic factor, vitamin B_{12} and the serum from a patient with this disease. The serum was found to prevent intrinsic factor from mediating the absorption of B_{12} into the body, and further studies showed the active principle to be an antibody. Antibody in the serum does not seem to be capable of neutralizing the physiological activity of intrinsic factor; a patient immunized parenterally with hog intrinsic factor in complete Freund's adjuvant had high serum antibody levels and good cell-mediated skin responses but still absorbed B_{12} well when fed with hog intrinsic factor. These data imply that the antibodies have to be present within the lumen of the gastro-intestinal tract to be biologically effective, and indeed they can be identified in the gastric juice of these patients, synthesized by plasma cells in the gastritic lesion.

Sperm

In some infertile males, agglutinating antibodies cause aggregation of the spermatozoa and interfere with their penetration into the cervical mucus.

Glomerular basement membrane (gbm)

With immunological kidney disease the experimental models preceded the finding of parallel lesions in the human. Injection of cross-reacting heterologous gbm preparations in complete Freund's adjuvant produces glomerulonephritis in sheep and other experimental animals. Antibodies to gbm can be picked up by immunofluorescent staining with anti-IgG of biopsies from nephritic animals. The antibodies are largely if not completely absorbed out by the kidney *in vivo* but they appear in the serum on nephrectomy and can passively transfer the disease to another animal of the same species.

An entirely analogous situation occurs in man in certain cases of glomerulonephritis, particularly those associated with lung haemorrhage (Goodpasture's syndrome). Kidney biopsy from the patient shows *linear* deposition of IgG and the β_{1C} component of complement along the basement membrane of the glomerular capillaries (figure 6.9a). After nephrectomy, gbm antibodies can be detected in the serum. Dixon and his colleagues eluted the gbm antibody from a diseased kidney and injected it into a squirrel monkey. The antibody rapidly fixed to the gbm of the recipient animal and produced a fatal nephritis (figure 9.12). It is hard to escape the conclusion that the lesion in the human was the direct result of attack on the gbm by

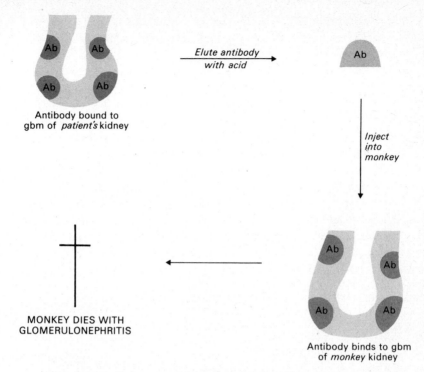

Antibody bound to
gbm of *patient's* kidney

Elute antibody
with acid

Ab

Inject
into
monkey

Ab

Ab

Ab

Ab

Antibody binds to gbm
of *monkey* kidney

MONKEY DIES WITH
GLOMERULONEPHRITIS

FIGURE 9.12. Passive transfer of glomerulonephritis to a squirrel monkey by injection of antiglomerular basement membrane (anti-gbm) antibodies isolated by acid elution from the kidney of a patient with Goodpasture's syndrome (after Lerner R.A., Glassock R.J. & Dixon F.J., *J.exp.Med.* 1967, **126**, 989).

these complement-fixing antibodies. The lung changes in Goodpasture's syndrome may be attributable to cross reaction with some of the gbm antibodies.

Table 9.4 summarizes these direct pathogenic effects of humoral autoantibodies.

EFFECTS OF COMPLEXES

Where autoantibodies are formed against soluble components to which they have continual access, complexes may be formed which can give rise to lesions similar to those occurring in serum sickness (cf. 145). In SLE, complexes of DNA and other nuclear antigens with immunoglobulin and complement can be detected in the kidneys of patients with evidence of renal dysfunction by immunofluorescent staining of biopsies. The staining pattern with a fluorescent anti-IgG or anti-β_{1C} (C3) is punctate or 'lumpy-bumpy' as some would describe it (figure 6.9b) in marked contrast with the linear pattern caused by the gbm antibodies in Goodpasture's syndrome (figure 6.9a; p. 140). The complexes grow in size to become large aggregates visible in the electron microscope as amorphous humps on the epithelial side of the glomerular basement membrane. During the active phase of the disease, serum complement levels fall as components are pulled out by these antigen–antibody aggregates in the kidney. Immunofluorescent studies on skin biopsies from patients with the related disease discoid lupus erythematosus also reveal the presence of immune complexes.

IgG in immune complexes can provoke the formation of autoantibodies—the so-called rheumatoid or antiglobulin factors—and these are demonstrable in the sera of virtually all patients with rheumatoid arthritis. The majority have IgM antiglobulins which react in the classical agglutination tests (p. 214, note 6). Seronegative patients who fail to react in these tests nonetheless can be shown to have elevated levels of IgG

TABLE 9.4. Direct pathogenic effects of humoral antibodies

Disease	Autoantigen	Lesion
Autoimmune haemolytic anaemia	Red cell	Erythrocyte destruction
Lymphopenia (some cases)	Lymphocyte	Lymphocyte destruction
Idiopathic thrombocytopenic purpura	Platelet	Platelet destruction
Male infertility (some cases)	Sperm	Agglutination of spermatozoa
Pernicious anaemia	Intrinsic factor	Neutralization of ability to mediate B_{12} absorption
Hashimoto's disease	Thyroid surface antigen	Cytotoxic effect on thyroid cells in culture
Thyrotoxicosis	? Thyroid surface antigen	Stimulation of thyroid cells
Goodpasture's syndrome	Glomerular basement membrane	Complement mediated damage to basement membrane

antiglobulins detectable by immunoadsorption techniques (cf. p. 107). In the light of this consistent evidence for sensitization to IgG it is relevant to note that aggregated IgG perhaps in the form of complexes can be detected in the synovium and the synovial fluid and polymorphs in the affected joints of patients with rheumatoid arthritis. Complement levels in the synovial fluid are low and soluble aggregates of IgG can be detected by precipitation reactions in agar with C1q and as complexes in cryoprecipitates (cf. p. 147). Ig, complement and rheumatoid factors can be demonstrated within the poly-morphs, and their phagocytosis leads to release of lysosomal enzymes which contribute to the inflammatory reaction within the joint. The synovium typically is very heavily infiltrated with mononuclear cells often aggregated in the form of lym-phoid follicles; there are many plasma cells and it has been estimated that the synthesis of IgG can be as high as that of a stimulated lymph node. Is IgG itself the only antigen respons-ible for evoking this response or is the synthesis of anti-globulin factors secondary to immune complex formation in-volving a quite separate antigen—say an endogenous joint constituent or an exogenous agent such as a micro-organism? To take just one of the many possibilities, infection with a number of mycoplasma strains is known to cause arthritis in a wide variety of different animal species; Williams has recently reported the isolation of *Mycoplasma fermentans* from the synovial fluids of patients with seropositive rheumatoid arthri-tis but confirmation is awaited. In addition to a humoral anti-body response which could give rise to immune complex-mediated hypersensitivity, a cellular hypersensitivity might also be involved and under these conditions it is known that intra-articular antigen can provoke a chronic arthritic reaction.

Certain Hashimoto sera contain a high molecular weight component (probably some form of thyroglobulin complex) which endows blood leucocytes from a normal subject with the ability to kill thyroglobulin coated chicken cells. This looks very much like some form of K-cell arming and it seems prob-able that a similar phenomenon underlies the ability of Hashi-moto leucocytes to kill thyroglobulin-coated target cells directly *in vitro*. So far as we know, thyroglobulin does not constitute part of the thyroid cell surface and we must be un-certain about a pathogenetic role for such armed cells. Perhaps they might react with thyroglobulin deposited (? as a complex) in the extrafollicular thyroid connective tissue to release tissue damaging factors?

CELL-MEDIATED HYPERSENSITIVITY

The inflammatory infiltrate in organ specific autoimmune disease is usually essentially mononuclear in character and, although not an infallible guide, this has been taken as an ex-pression of cell-mediated hypersensitivity. Direct evidence is still thin. At the time of writing, skin reactions to autoantigens have proved difficult to assess and *in vitro* leucocyte inhibition tests have not been unequivocally accepted although for example in autoimmune thyroiditis and thyrotoxicosis there is a consistent finding of inhibition of leucocyte migration by thyroid microsomes. The killing of colon cells in culture by lymphocytes from patients with ulcerative colitis is encouraging and it has been reported that long-term culture of thyroid target cells with Hashimoto leucocytes leads to significant failure in the metabolic handling of iodine. Firm evidence for a direct participation of T-lymphocytes in any of these reactions has yet to be provided. Indirect evidence for a destructive role

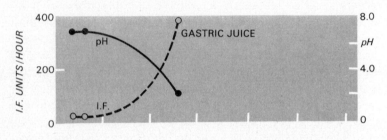

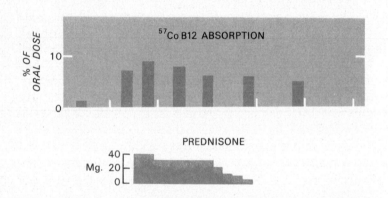

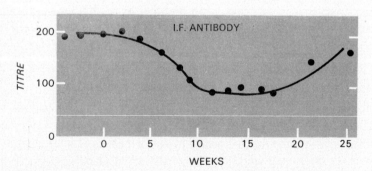

FIGURE 9.13. Regeneration of gastric mucosal function in pernicious anaemia after steroid treatment (from Ardeman S. & Chanarin I., *N.Engl.J.Med.* 1965, **273**, 1352).

234

of the inflammatory cells comes from the observation that high doses of steroids may restore gastric function in certain patients with pernicious anaemia. In one such case studied, biopsy after intensive treatment with prednisone showed diminution in cellular infiltrate and new formation of parietal and chief cells in the gastric mucosa; acid and intrinsic factor were now produced after histamine stimulation and the ability to absorb vitamin B_{12} assessed by the Schilling test was restored to near normal values (figure 9.13). The most likely explanation is that attack by the inflammatory cells and attempts to regenerate by mucosal cells were more or less in balance in the atrophic mucosa. Elimination of inflammatory cells by the prednisone allowed the regeneration of gastric mucosal cells to become evident.

Our views on the pathogenesis of pernicious anaemia may be stated as follows. Autoimmune attack based on the parietal cell antigen gives rise to an atrophic gastritis which in many cases settles down to a dynamic equilibrium where the rate of destruction roughly balances the rate of regeneration; the loss of capacity to make intrinsic factor is evident in tests showing defective B_{12} absorption but sufficient vitamin is absorbed to keep the body in balance. These patients often have parietal cell antibodies and go on for 15 years or so without developing megaloblastic anaemia. However, if they should produce antibodies to intrinsic factor in the lumen of the gastrointestinal tract, these will neutralize the small amount of intrinsic factor still available and the body will move into negative balance for B_{12}. The symptoms of B_{12} deficiency will then appear some considerable time later as the liver stores become exhausted (figure 9.14).

The nature of the cellular attack in organ-specific disorders is still not resolved but it is not improbable that cell-mediated hypersensitivity, direct antibody cytotoxicity and inflammatory reactions due to immune complexes may operate alone or in concert.

EXPERIMENTAL MODELS OF
AUTOIMMUNE DISEASE

If autoimmune processes are pathogenic in human diseases we would expect that the production of autoimmunity should lead to comparable lesions in experimental animals.

Experimental autoallergic disease

When animals are injected with extracts of certain organs emulsified in oil containing killed tubercle bacilli (i.e. in complete Freund's adjuvant), autoantibodies and destructive inflammatory lesions specific to the organ used for immunization result. Thus, Rose and Witebsky found that rabbits receiving rabbit thyroglobulin in Freund's adjuvant developed antibodies to thyroglobulin and thyroiditis involving invasion of the gland by mononuclear cells of lymphocytic and histiocytic types with destruction of the normal follicular architecture. Histologically there are many points of similarity between this experimental autoallergic lesion and human autoimmune thyroiditis as seen in Hashimoto's disease and primary myxoedema (figure 9.15).

In some of the earliest work in this field it was shown that injection of central nervous tissue produced encephalomyelitis and paralysis in monkeys and guinea-pigs; the parallel with post rabies vaccine encephalitis is clear since the vaccine contains brain extracts, and optimistic comparisons with multiple sclerosis have been made. Similarly lesions can be induced in the adrenal (cf. Addisonian idiopathic adrenal atrophy), the testis (? model for granulomatous orchitis) and stomach (cf.

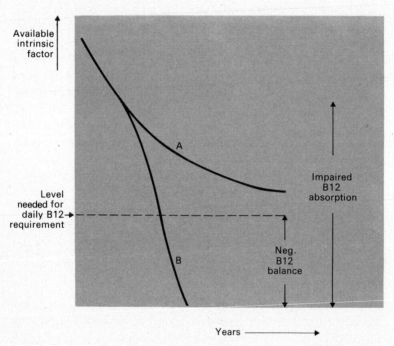

FIGURE 9.14. Pathogenesis of pernicious anaemia. Group A: Patients with long standing atrophic gastritis having parietal cell but no intrinsic factor antibodies. Group B: Pernicious anaemia patients with intrinsic factor antibodies superimposed upon the atrophic gastritis. (After Doniach D. & Roitt I.M., *Seminars in Hematology* 1964, **1**, 313.)

atrophic gastritis of pernicious anaemia). Heterologous glomeruli stimulate the formation of glomerular basement membrane autoantibodies which localize in the kidney of the host to cause severe glomerulonephritis (Steblay model) resembling closely that seen in Goodpasture's syndrome.

The experimental disease can usually be transmitted to syngeneic animals by lymphoid cells from immunized donors and occasionally by serum. In the case of experimental autoallergic orchitis, a synergism between cell-mediated hypersensitivity and antibody was recognized in the transfer studies.

Abnormalities of neuromuscular conduction resembling those seen in myasthenia gravis together with muscle autoantibodies can be evoked in guinea-pigs by muscle or thymus in Freund's adjuvant. Because these neuromuscular changes were *not* observed when the same experiments were carried out in thymectomized adults even though similar antibodies were formed, Goldberg put forward the view, independently supported by histological observations, that the fundamental lesion in myasthenia is an autoimmune reaction with the thymus as a target, releasing a soluble factor which acts as an inhibitor of neuromuscular conduction.

Although the precise nature of the events leading to tissue damage have yet to be resolved, it is abundantly clear that the deliberate provocation of an autoallergic state can produce lesions which closely mimic those seen in human organ specific autoimmune disease and add weight to the notion that the immunological events are directly concerned in the pathogenesis of these disorders.

Spontaneous autoimmune disease

A strain of chickens has been found to develop thyroiditis with thyroglobulin autoantibodies leading to eventual thyroid deficiency. These changes could be prevented by neonatal bursectomy but not thymectomy, suggesting the possibility that the thyroid antibodies were primarily involved in the production of the tissue lesions.

The now famous strain of mouse, the New Zealand Black (NZB), consistently develops an autoimmune haemolytic anaemia with positive Coombs' tests (agglutination of antibody coated erythrocytes by an antiglobulin serum). The disease can be provoked in young unaffected NZB's by transfer of spleen cells from a Coombs' positive donor showing that it is the production of red cell antibodies which leads to shortened

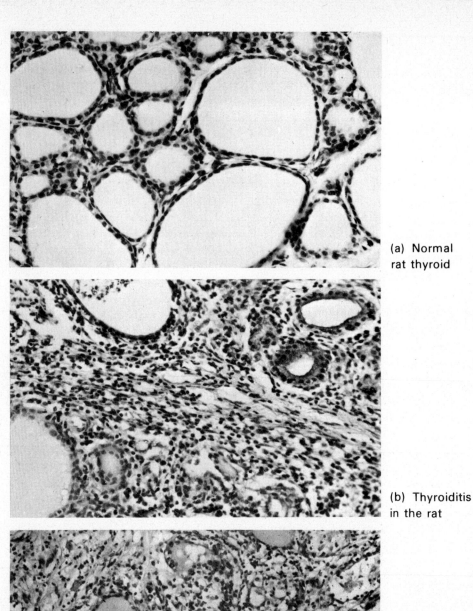

(a) Normal
rat thyroid

(b) Thyroiditis
in the rat

(c) Hashimoto's
disease

erythrocyte survival and consequent anaemia. A high proportion of these mice, and especially their hybrids with the partially related New Zealand White (B × W F1), have circulating antinuclear antibodies, may give a positive LE-cell test (cf. SLE p. 217) and have an immune complex induced glomerulonephritis. The kidney disease can be transferred to unaffected young NZB mice with lymphoid cells (particularly when the recipients are first immunosuppressed) and it seems certain that these lesions are immunologically induced. Virus particles are regularly seen in the tissues and it has been suggested that they are responsible for the high incidence of lymphoid tumours in these mice and for the production of autoantibodies; the kidney complexes contain DNA and viral antigen is present cf. p. 225.

Diagnostic value of autoantibody tests

Serum autoantibodies frequently provide valuable diagnostic markers. The most useful routine test is screening of the serum by immunofluorescence on a composite unfixed frozen section of thyroid, stomach and kidney. This is supplemented by agglutination tests for thyroglobulin and red cell antibodies and rheumatoid factors, by complement fixation, by radioassay for intrinsic factor antibodies and so on (see table 9.2). The salient information is summarized in table 9.5.

The tests will also prove of value in screening for people at risk, e.g. relatives of patients with autoimmune disease, thyroiditis patients (for gastric autoimmunity and *vice versa*) and ultimately the general population.

Treatment of autoimmune disorders

In cases of organ-specific disease, replacement therapy is usually adequate, e.g. thyroxine in primary myxoedema, vitamin B_{12} in pernicious anaemia and so forth.

In SLE and immune complex nephritis, steroids, often in high doses, help to suppress the inflammatory lesions. Attempts are made to inhibit the synthesis of autoantibodies by immunosuppressive drugs such as azathioprine, cyclophosphamide and

FIGURE 9.15. Similarity of lesions in Hashimoto's disease of the human and experimental autoallergic thyroiditis produced by injection of rats with homologous thyroid in complete Freund's adjuvant.

TABLE 9.5. Autoantibody tests and diagnosis

Disease	Antibody	Comment
Hashimoto's thyroiditis	Thyroid	Distinction from colloid goitre, thyroid cancer and subacute thyroiditis Thyroidectomy usually unnecessary in Hashimoto goitre
Primary myxoedema	Thyroid	Tests +ve in 99 per cent of cases. If suspected hypothyroidism assess 'thyroid reserve' by TSH stimulation test
Thyrotoxicosis	Thyroid	High titres esp. CFT indicate active thyroiditis and tendency to post-operative myxoedema: anti-thyroid drugs treatment of choice
Pernicious anaemia	Stomach	Help in diagnosis of latent P.A. in differential diagnosis of non-auto-immune megaloblastic anaemia and in suspected subacute combined degeneration of the cord
Idiopathic adrenal atrophy	Adrenal	Distinction from tuberculous form
Myasthenia gravis	Muscle	When positive suggests associated thymoma
Pemphigus vulgaris and pemphigoid	Skin	Different fluorescent patterns in the two diseases
Autoimmune haemolytic anaemia	Erythrocyte (Coombs' test)	Distinction from other forms of anaemia
Sjögren's syndrome	Salivary duct cells	
Primary biliary cirrhosis (PBC)	Mitochondrial	Distinction from other forms of obstructive jaundice where test rarely +ve Recognize subgroup within cryptogenic cirrhosis related to PBC with +ve mitochondrial Ab
Active chronic hepatitis	Smooth muscle anti-nuclear and 20 per cent mitochondrial	Smooth muscle Ab distinguish from SLE
Rheumatoid arthritis	Antiglobulin, e.g. SCAT and latex fixation	High titre indicative of bad prognosis
SLE	High titre antinuclear, DNA; LE-cells	DNA antibodies present in active phase
Scleroderma	Nucleolar	
Other 'collagenoses'	Nuclear	

methotrexate. Long-term treatment with anti-lymphocyte serum is still considered hazardous and uncertain in outcome.

In rheumatoid arthritis anti-inflammatory drugs such as aspirin are extensively used. If micro-organisms can be convincingly implicated in the pathogenesis of this disease then they will become the natural chemotherapeutic target.

Further reading

Doniach D., Walker J.G., Roitt I.M. & Berg P.A. (1970) Autoallergic hepatitis. *N. Eng. J. Med.* **282**, 86.

Gell P.G.H., Coombs R.R.A. & Lachmann P. (eds.) (1974) Clinical Aspects of Immunology, 3rd ed. Blackwell Scientific Publications, Oxford

Glynn L.E. & Holborow E.J. (1964) *Autoimmunity and Disease.* Blackwell Scientific Publications, Oxford

Miescher P.A. & Grabar P. (eds) *Series of International Symposia on Immunopathology.* Schwabe & Co., Basle.

Miescher P.A. & Muller-Eberhard H.J. (eds) (1968) *Textbook of Immunopathology.* Grune & Stratton, New York

Roitt I.M. & Doniach D. (1967) Delayed hypersensitivity in autoimmune disease. *Brit. med. Bull.* 23, 66.

Samter M. (ed) (1971) *Immunological Diseases.* Little Brown, New York

Turk J.L. (1973) *Immunology in Clinical Medicine.* Heinemann, London

Weigle W.O. (1971) Recent observations and concepts in immunological unresponsiveness and autoimmunity. *Clin. Exp. Immunol.* **9**, 437

Zvaifler H.J. (1973) The immunopathology of joint inflammation in rheumatoid arthritis. *Advances in Immunology.* **16**, 265.

Summary: comparison of organ-specific and non-organ-specific diseases

Organ-specific (e.g. Thyroiditis, Gastritis, Adrenalitis)	Non-organ specific (e.g. Systemic Lupus Erythematosus
Differences	
1. Antigens only available to lymphoid system in low concentration and immune tolerance not firmly established	Antigens fully accessible and tolerance established normally
2. Antibodies organ-specific	Antibodies non-organ-specific
3. Clinical and serologic overlap— thyroiditis, gastritis and adrenalitis	Overlap SLE, rheumatoid arthritis, and other connective tissue disorders
4. Familial tendency to organ-specific autoimmunity	Familial connective tissue disease ? Abnormalities in immuno-globulin synthesis in relatives
5. Therapy aimed at replacing specific hormones	Therapy aimed at inhibiting inflammation and antibody synthesis
6. Lymphoid invasion, parenchymal destruction by ? ± cell mediated hypersensitivity ? ± antibodies	Lesions due to deposition antigen–antibody complexes
7. Antigens evoke antibodies in normal animals with complete Freund's adjuvant	No antibodies produced in animals with comparable stimulation
8. Experimental lesions produced with antigen in Freund adjuvant	Diseases and autoantibodies arise spontaneously in certain animals (e.g. NZB mice and hybrids and some dogs) or after injection of parental lymphoid tissue into F1 hybrids

Similarities

1. Circulating autoantibodies react with normal body constituents
2. Patients often have increased immunoglobulins in serum
3. Antibodies may appear in each of the main immunoglobulin classes
4. Greater incidence in women
5. Disease process not always progressive; exacerbations and remissions
6. Autoantibody tests of diagnostic value

Appendix

Ministry of Health schedule of vaccination and immunization procedures

Age	Prophylactic	Interval
During the first year of life	Diph/Tet/Pert and oral Polio vaccine (First dose)	
Note The earliest age at which the first dose should be given is 3 months, but a better general immunological response can be expected if the first dose is delayed to 6 months of age.	Diph/Tet/Pert and oral Polio vaccine (Second dose) Diph/Tet/Pert and oral Polio vaccine (Third dose)	Preferably after an interval of 6–8 weeks Preferably after an interval of 6 months
During the second year of life	Measles vaccination	After an interval of not less than 3 weeks (see note 9)
At 5 years of age or school entry *Note* These may be given, if desired, at 3 years of age to children entering nursery schools, attending day nurseries or living in children's homes.	Diph/Tet and oral Polio vaccine or Diph/Tet/Polio vaccine	
Between 10 and 13 years of age (see note 10) Girls 11–14 years of age	BCG vaccine (for tuberculin-negative children) Rubella vaccination	
At 15–19 years of age or on leaving school	Polio vaccine (oral or inactivated) Tetanus toxoid	

Additional notes

1. The basic course of immunization against diphtheria, pertussis, tetanus and poliomyelitis should be completed at as early an age as possible consistent with the likelihood of a good immunological response. Live measles vaccine should not be given to children below the age of 9 months, since it usually fails to immunize such children owing to the presence of maternally transmitted antibodies.

Reinforcement of immunization against diphtheria, tetanus and poliomyelitis should be undertaken at about the age of first entry to school.

Further reinforcement of immunization against tetanus and poliomyelitis should be offered at school leaving age.

2. Examples of timing of doses of basic course of immunization:

	1st dose	*2nd dose*	*3rd dose*
Age	3 months	5 months	9–12 months
	4 ,,	6 ,,	10–12 ,,
	5 ,,	7 ,,	about 12 months
	6 ,,	8 ,,	about 12–14 months
	Interval	Interval	
	6–8 weeks	Preferably 6, and not less than 4, months	

3. The desirable commencing age for immunization is 6 months of age because (a) before this age the antibody response may be reduced by the presence of maternal antibody, (b) the child's antibody-forming mechanism is immature in the early months of life, and (c) severe reactions to pertussis vaccine are less common in children over 6 months old than at 3 months of age.

4. The boosting dose of triple vaccine previously recommended to be given during the second year is considered to be unnecessary if the three-dose schedule spaced as in (2) is followed.

5. If no immunization, or an incomplete basic course of immunization, has been given before school entry the full basic course of diphtheria, tetanus, pertussis and poliomyelitis immunization should be given at school entry, but vaccination against smallpox should not be undertaken unless a need arises (see note 7).

6. The boosting dose of diphtheria and tetanus toxoid previously recommended to be given at 8 to 12 years of age is considered in the light of accumulating information to be unnecessary if the three-dose schedule space as in (2) is followed and a booster dose given at 5 years of age or school entry. A booster dose of tetanus toxoid alone is recommended at 15 to 19 years of age or on leaving school.

7. Vaccination is a safe and reliable method of protection against smallpox for the vast majority of persons but the number of serious complications in childhood, though few, is now out of proportion to the risk from smallpox in Britain. Thus vaccination against smallpox need no longer be recommended as a routine procedure in early childhood. All travellers to and from areas of the world where smallpox is endemic or countries where

eradication programmes are in progress should be protected by recent vaccination. Although primary vaccination in adult life also carries a risk of complications, recently compiled data indicate that this is not so great as to justify routine vaccination in childhood in the hope of reducing the risk to adults. Past experience has shown that health service staff are particularly liable to be exposed to infection after an importation of smallpox and the importance of the vaccination and regular re-vaccination of all health service staff who come into contact with patients is emphasized. When considering the need for vaccination or re-vaccination due attention should be paid to the known contra-indications.

8. In view of the possibility of accidental infection of eczematous members of the family of a child vaccinated against smallpox it would be preferable for all routine smallpox vaccinations to be carried out by or with the knowledge of the family doctor.

9. An interval of 3 to 4 weeks should normally be allowed to elapse between the administration of any two live vaccines or between the administration of diphtheria/tetanus/pertussis vaccine and a live vaccine, other than oral poliomyelitis vaccine, whichever is given first.

10. Whereas the normal age for BCG vaccination is during the year preceding the fourteenth birthday, the local epidemiological situation may sometimes call for early BCG vaccination. A local health authority may therefore, at their discretion, vaccinate school children aged 10 years or more if in their view this appears to be justified. In certain areas BCG vaccine is given as a routine in infancy.

11. Because the foetus is so vulnerable to rubella in the first trimester of pregnancy, it is desirable to immunize girls before child-bearing age. Routine rubella vaccination of women of child-bearing age is not recommended. However, any women who have been tested during pregnancy for rubella antibodies and have been found to be seronegative should be offered rubella vaccine in the early post-partum period. School teachers may be exposed to a greater risk of natural infection in the classroom and nurses in children's hospitals and obstetric units are at special risk because they may come in contact with babies suffering from congenital rubella. Staff working in antenatal clinics may, if they become naturally infected, transmit rubella to patients who may be in the early stages of pregnancy. Individuals in these groups should have their antibody status determined and those found to be seronegative should be offered vaccination.

245

Index

Antibody *(cont.)*
  -forming cells 46, 65
  heterologous 173
  homologous 173
  homocytotropic 129, 133, 171
  humoral *see* Humoral antibody
  interaction with antigen *in vitro*
    99–126
  level tests *see* Antigen binding
    techniques
  production 1
    in transplantation 183
  reaginic *see* homocytotropic
  response to antigen 1
    primary 43–4
    regulation of 71
    secondary 44–6
  serum 168
  site 17
  specificity 16, 29
  synthesis 43–80
    in relation to cell-mediated
      hypersensitivity 153
    theories of 83–98
  variability, genetic theories of
    94–8
Antigen (Ag) 1
  absence from plasma cells 84
  -antibody
    binding 8–12
    techniques 106–9
  dosage 89
  excess (AgXS), (serum sickness)
    125, 145
  interaction with antibody *in vitro*
    99–126
  -sensitive cells, detection of
    65–8
  -specific depression of homograft
    reactivity 200
  thymus-dependent 72, 78
  thymus-independent 62
  wells 105
Antigenic
  competition 71
  determinants 4, 17
  variation 170–1
Antigenicity
  relevance to, of co-operation
    between B- and T-cells 61
Antiglobulin coprecipitation
    technique 106
Anti-light chains 58

Antilymphocyte
  globulin (ALG) 196–9
  serum (ALS) 157
Anti-ovalbumin 5
Antiserum 12, 14, 15
Appendix 49
Arsonates 8
Arthus reaction 142, 144
Aspartate 9, 10
Aspirin 241
Asthma 39
Ataxia telengiectasia 178, 179
Atopic allergy 39, 134–5
Atrophic gastritis, autoimmune
  212, 219, 242
Australia antigen *see* Hepatitis B
  (Australia) antigen
Autoallergic
  disease, experimental 235
  orchitis, experimental 237
Autoantibodies 2
  diagnostic value of tests for 239
  in human disease 212–17
  incidence in general population
    221
  intrinsic factor 213, 214, 229–30
  production of 80
Autograft 181
Autoimmune
  atrophic gastritis 212, 219, 242
  disease
    experimental models of 235
    genetic factors of 219
    pathogenic mechanisms in
      spontaneous 237 [226–39
    treatment of 239–41
  haemolytic anaemia 212, 219
    associated with administration
      of chlorpromazine 141
      α-methyl dopa 223
      phenacetin 141
    autoantibodies in 139, 213
    autoantibody tests and diag-
      nosis 240
    cytotoxic reactions in 125
    humoral antibodies in 232
    opsonic adherence in 116
  reactions: in cytotoxic-type
    hypersensitivity 139
  response 221
Autoimmunity 211–41
Avidity 15, 90, 91, 114
Azathioprine 196, 202, 239

Drugs
  cytotoxic 179
  immunosuppressive 195–6,
    239, 241
  reactions to 141

Earthworm: phylogeny of immunity
  74
Eczema 178, 245
Effector cells 44
Egg albumin 132
Electron cloud shape 8, 11, 12, 14
Electrophoresis
  crossover 102, 104
  paper 72
  rocket 103, 105 (fig. 5.6)
  separation of B- and T-cells by
    57
see also Immunoelectrophoresis
Encephalitis 175, 223, 236
Endocytosis 58, 113
Endosmosis 104
Endotoxin 39, 62, 64, 121, 122
  shock 125
Enhancement 200–2
Enzyme basis of amplifying com-
    plement cascade 118
Epitopes 4
Epstein-Barr (EB) virus 206
Erythema 142–3, 148
Escherichia coli 124 (fig. 5.23),
    224
Exotoxins 174

Farmer's lung 125, 145
Farr technique 106, 107 (fig. 5.8)
Ferritin 113
First set reactions 181–2, 197
Flagellin
  polymerized 88
  radioactive salmonella 88
Fluorescein 58, 65, 109, 111, 113
Fluorescent
  antibody tests see Immuno-
    fluorescent test (IFT)
  dyes
    fluorescein 58, 65, 109, 111,
      113
    rhodamine 109
Focus formation 68

Foetal-maternal immunological re-
    lationship 209
α-foetoprotein 204, 207
Formaldehyde 174
Fractionation 22 (fig. 2.2), 23
Fragment
  antigen binding (Fab) 22, 33,
    57, 58, 85
  crystallizable (Fc) 22, 26, 33,
    34, 56, 59, 61, 197
Freund's adjuvant
  complete 153, 154, 167, 223,
    230, 236
    mode of action 70–1
  incomplete 175

β-galactosidase 117, 157
Gastric parietal cells 110–11
Gastritis, atrophic, autoimmune
    212, 219, 242
Gel filtration 22 (fig. 2.2), 23
Genetic
  markers 41, 95
  studies in antibody synthesis 85
  theories of antibody variability
    94–8
Germ line theory 94
Gershon's infectious tolerance 78
see also Immunological tolerance
γ-globulin 21, 27
  as prophylactic 173
  treatment of B-cell deficiency
    176
Glomerular basement membrane
    (gbm) 230
Glomerulonephritis 125, 140, 202,
    230
Glutamyl 85
Glutaraldehyde 107
Glycines 14
Glycoproteins 184
Goodpasture's syndrome 202, 212
  autoantibodies in 213
  gbm antibodies in 139, 230, 231,
    232
  humoral antibodies in 232
Grafts
  cartilage 202
  clincial experience in 202–4
  corneal 202
  heart 202
  kidney 202

251

T-lymphocytes (thymus-dependent) 48
  activity related to hypersensitivity and immunity 154
  co-operation with B-lymphocytes 59–65
  deficiency in children 176–7
  function inhibited by ALG 198
  identification 49, 55
  in immunological tolerance 78–80, 93
  mediating specific immunity 165
  response in lowliest vertebrates 75
  rosette formation in 66
Tannic acid 114
Tears: IgA antibodies in 163
Tetanus 65
  bacillus
    chemical modification 174
  vaccination against 243, 244, 245
  with γ-globulin 173
Theophylline 229
Thoracic duct cannulation 195
Thrombocytopenia 178
  neonatal 226
Thrombocytopenic purpura, idiopathic (ITP) 141, 212, 213, 219, 226, 232
Thrush *see* Candida albicans
Thymectomy
  adult 57, 71, 80
  neonatal
    effect of, on development of immunological competence 46, 47, 59
    effect of, on skin grafts 182
    similarity to T-cell deficiency 177
Thymic
  dysplasias 49
  hypoplasias 176
Thymocytes 60, 79
Thymosin 46
Thymus 46–7, 73
  -dependent antigens 72, 78
  in fish 75
  graft 176
  -independent antigens 62
  removal of *see* Thymectomy
Thyroglobulin 4, 222

Thyroid 226–9
  -stimulating hormone (TSH) 126, 155, 222, 228, 229
Thyroiditis 227, 242
  Hashimoto's *see* Hashimoto's disease
Thyrotoxicosis 212
  autoantibodies in 213
  autoantibody tests and diagnosis 240
  humoral antibodies in 232
  thyroid stimulation in 227
Thyroxine 229, 239
Tissue
  culture 59, 93
  damage 154–5
  matching 193–4
  storage banks 194
  transplants 130
  typing in man 186–8
Titre (definition) 115
Tobacco mosaic virus (TMV) protein 17
Tolerance *see* Immunological tolerance
Tonsil 49
Toxoids: in active immunization 174
Toxoplasma goudii 171
Transferrin 9, 103
Transfusion reactions 137
Transplantation 181–210
  antigens 139, 183–8
  reactions: small lymphocytes in 44
Trichinella spiralis 171
Tri-iodothyronine 229
Trophoblast 210
Trypanosomiasis 170
Trypsin 122, 227
Tryptophan 9
Tubercle bacillus 165, 179
Tuberculosis 154
Tumours
  epithelial 179
  liver 102
  lymphoid system 179
Typhoid 174
Tyrosine 85

Ulcerative colitis 212, 214, 224
Uraemia 202

Tra~~ facto K9~~

259